A WARRIOR'S DEATH

Volume 2 in A Byzantine
Murder Mystery

M.L. Jerinic

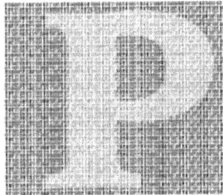

Palamedes

San Francisco

Palamedes Publishing
www.palamedes.pub
San Francisco

Cover by Katarina Jerinic
www.katarinajerinic.com

Cover image: *Panel from an Ivory Casket with the Killing of the King of Hazor (Joshua 11)*, Byzantine, 10th-11th century, Metropolitan Museum of Art, Open Access (CC0)

ISBN 978-0-9996930-2-5
LCCN 2024949437

Also available in ebook:
EPUB 5f906878-4d76-4224-81bc-1e73e1a897cf
www.palamedes.pub/books/warriors-death

www.facebook.com/PalamedesPub
www.twitter.com/PalamedesPub
www.instagram.com/PalamedesPub

Dedication

For those who have gone before us, Memory Eternal.

Chapter 1

November 10, 1047
Near the Walls of Constantinople

H*e had arrived, but he dared not let down his guard—not yet.*
Like the shadowy bulk of a mountain range, the walls of Constantinople rose before him in the moonlight. He slowed his horse with a tug on the reins, and the clatter of his mount's iron-clad hooves diminished. They struck the paving stones of the Adrianople road in a deliberate, measured cadence. And now even the chill north wind that had lashed his face and howled throughout the journey had died down. He found the night uncomfortably quiet.

He veered left off the broad way and headed northward, towards Blachernae Palace. At that moment, a light flared on one of the towers of the wall. One sentry called out to another, but his words could not be distinguished.

In no time, he reached a postern gate in the very shadow of the Palace. Up on the wall, someone appeared with a lantern. "Halt!"

Down below, he reined in.

"The password," came the voice from above.

"'The truth shall make you free.'" The phrase had been assigned to him before he set out. How appropriate it had proved to be!

"Enter." Something rattled and clanked on the other side of the gate, and the iron-studded door creaked open.

He entered the passageway, and as the clip-clop of his horse's hooves echoed against the walls, a sweat broke out on his back.

A soldier stationed inside the wall saluted him. "Welcome back, sir."

"Thank you," he said, bowing in the saddle.

"Why so late?"

"I couldn't avoid it."

"You're bound for the Great Palace now?"

"Yes." He had news that would make the Court tremble.

As the gate clanked shut behind him, he turned his horse onto a side street leading south to the Mese, Constantinople's main thoroughfare. Within minutes he passed the glossy waters of a cistern that mirrored the moonlit sky.

On both sides of the street, the land sloped away into shadows. This part of the City was sparsely populated and largely occupied by vineyards, fields, and pastures.

Ahead, far along the ridge, the five gold domes of the Church of the Holy Apostles gleamed pale. His heart lifted at the sight.

Still, he was in no hurry to reach his destination. When he had traversed about half a mile, he slowed his horse to a walk and peered into the darkness to his right. A short way down the hill loomed a stone building: an abandoned barn, with the purple night sky showing through the black ribs of its ruined roof.

This was the place. Now—or at least after tonight, he could dispose of the matter.

He turned his horse towards the barn, conscious of the

faint babble of voices that drifted towards him from the east, from deeper in the City. He looked in the direction of the noise and saw warm yellow light seeping out into the gloom—from around closed shutters. No doubt it was a tavern staying open after hours, or even worse—a bordello. It was bad that tavern-keepers flouted the law to stay open, and even worse that no officials thought to close the brothels.

Clenching the leather-wrapped hilt of the dagger at his belt, he rode around the barn, glaring into the black maw of the doorway. Had something moved there?

"Hello?" he called.

His horse nickered.

Something rustled behind him, and he turned quickly.

He faced only a clump of trees and underbrush. "Who goes there?"

Then a strange force seized him, tearing him from the saddle. He cried out. He kicked free of the stirrups. He tried to push himself free but could not overcome the thing constraining him.

"Fight!" he told himself, as he fell into darkness.

Chapter 2

Early the next morning, as the sky lightened into flaming orange above the golden domes of the Holy Apostles to the east, two farmers put their cows out on the slopes between the River Lycus and the Mese.

At once their muscular, short-haired herd dogs began to bark.

"Stop yer yawping!" yelled the graybeard Bartholomew.

The dogs did not stop but left their bovine charges and dashed for a beech grove about halfway up the hill.

"Back!" yelled their master. Instead, the dogs dove into the trees, growling and barking.

Cosmas, Bartholomew's black-bearded son, quickened his pace. "There's someone in there, Father, someone who doesn't belong."

Bartholomew watched the steamy plume of his son's breath. "Should I go back and get my bow?"

Cosmas wished he'd brought his own weapon, though he doubted they'd need it. He believed that the walls of Constantinople protected him from all dire perils. "Don't bother. Maybe it's just a rabbit. If it's anything bad, we can get the police."

"Yes, there must be a militiaman up on the street."

Cosmas loped up the incline. While the cows munched placidly on the drying grass, the old man tried to match his stride.

When Cosmas reached the grove, he pricked up his ears, but heard only the dogs' racket.

"Son, wait—"

Cosmas waved his father away and crashed into the trees, snapping small branches, crushing twigs and fallen leaves. He stopped short when he saw the dogs prancing around something formless and still, snapping furiously. "What the—"

Then, in the sunlight that angled in through the dense, newly-bare branches, he saw a man sprawled face down in the underbrush.

"*Kyrie eleison!* Lord, have mercy! He must be—"

Bartholomew charged in across the bed of leaves, then froze. Like his son, he gaped: a tall, well-proportioned figure, lay prone before him. A heavy cloak was twisted around his whitish tunic and fine wool hose.

Cosmas shouted above the frenzied barking. "Yes, he must be—"

His father patted the dogs' heads and scratched them between the ears. "Good work. Now git!" Once they were gone, he knelt beside the stranger and reached under him to feel his brow. "He's cold."

He cradled the man in his arms and turned him completely over, noting his fine aquiline nose. His hair and beard had been skillfully cut, despite their present disarray. "A gentleman!"

Bartholomew noticed that the dead man's dark eyes were flecked with red. Instinctively, he tried to close them.

"You'd better leave that for the militia," said Cosmas. "Maybe we shouldn't touch him."

"But this isn't decent," said the old man. Still, he abandoned his efforts almost immediately. "Mother of God, save us!" he exclaimed, crossing himself. I can't do it. He's getting stiff."

Cosmas turned on his heels, rustling the fallen leaves. "I'm going for the militia!" He dashed up the hill to the street, howling for help.

Some minutes later, he returned with two militiamen armed with spears and clubs. They burst into the wood, with Cosmas close behind them. Bartholomew managed a quick bow, then stepped aside. "I moved him. We found him on his stomach, but I wanted to close his eyes."

One of the militiamen had knelt down to examine the body. "He's dead all right, cold as the snows of Mt. Olympus! And he was murdered for certain. Strangled!" He indicated a thin red line around the victim's neck.

The other militiaman glanced a flash of sunlight off the dead man's right hand—a signet ring. He too knelt and examined the seal on the bezel. "Wait!" he said. "This is business for the Palace. This man was an agent of the Post."

Chapter 3

Back in the center of the City, in a modest house near the Forum of Constantine, Michael Taronites took a last look at himself in the battered bronze mirror on the wall. His beard was neatly combed, his lank dark hair in place. He looked respectable enough, except for the circles under his eyes. Once more he splashed cold water on his face. A lingering fatigue weighted his eyelids and bowed his shoulders.

He was about to go downstairs when he heard a hesitant knock on the door.

"Master?" it was George, his middle-aged manservant.

"Come in." Michael inclined his head to one side, curious. After last night's events, what did George have to say to him?

The servant pushed open the door, then bowed stiffly. "It's about Stephen, my boy." He looked up into Michael's eyes.

Michael's glance met the older man's eyes. He hid an ironic smile behind his hand. The "boy" in question was a few years older than Michael.

"Asleep, down in our rooms."

Michael nodded, not at all surprised. Stephen, George's son, had turned up roaring drunk last night, after being dismissed from his employment in the house of a leading family of the Empire. The "boy" could hardly have picked a worse time if he had wished to; Michael had just returned from a two-week journey.

"What will the whelp do now?" asked George.

"You'd like me to help him find another place."

George scratched his graying beard and looked down at his boots. "Yes."

Michael headed for his desk in the corner. "I'll write him a recommendation, since it's hardly prudent for him to use the name of his former employer."

"The man's a tyrant!"

"A tyrant?" Once seated, Michael opened the side compartment of his desk and took out a pen and an inkpot. "Isaac Comnenus is a soldier, an honest man but a hard one. As commander-in-chief of the eastern armies, he has little tolerance for...laxity." In other words, for tippling and sleeping on the job. George had similar weaknesses, but since he managed to get things done eventually, Michael overlooked them.

"Tell me," said Michael, as he inked his pen, "what sort of work did he do?"

"Maintenance, inside and out. Some gardening."

Using a fresh parchment leaf, Michael wrote in a neat, rounded hand that would have won the approval of most scribes and copyists. "Let him take this today—to the Palace—to the Rector or Head of the Imperial Household," he said, as he set down the finished document and sanded it. "From what I've heard, the man is no harsh taskmaster."

When the parchment was ready, George bowed again. "I thank you."

Michael felt a flush of embarrassment on his neck as he handed over the letter. "It's nothing," he said. But though he dismissed the favor with a wave of his hand, he was well aware that just three months ago, he lacked the confidence to perform such services. Nor would the authorities, have valued his opinion.

"Again, I thank you... Now I'll see to your horse."

Michael gave the servant a head start, then descended the wooden staircase into the rear hall. There he took his brown wool cloak from a peg. Bending his neck slightly, he stepped out into the pale sunlight that inundated the yard.

"Your horse is ready, Master."

"Thank you." Michael glanced up at the sun, which was almost halfway to the zenith. It was third hour of the day. "I'll be late, "he remarked, more to himself than to the servant.

George scratched his stomach. "Sorry about the disturbance last night. And I'm sorry I didn't get you up earlier."

"That wasn't your fault. I overslept. I was more worn out than I thought."

Worn out, or simply disappointed? Last night Michael had returned from the Anatolian city of Brusa, where, in his new capacity as an agent of the Post, he investigated discrepancies in postal workers' accounts and discovered that certain stationmasters were requisitioning State horses and carriages for their private use. Michael had arrested the culprits and arranged for supposedly honest men to replace them. It had been very straightforward work.

Still, he had expected more challenging work in his new position. The Post was, after, all, the governmental department of communications, foreign affairs, and state security. Both ordinary citizens and government officials stood in awe of it.

His hopes were not unreasonable—not for someone who had completely reversed the course of his life—if he had in fact done so. Slightly over two months ago, when he was a very minor official in the Imperial chancery, he had been accused of murdering the toady who had ruined his late father's life. But in a week's time he had unmasked the real killer and performed and rendered an invaluable service to the Empire.

He had been rewarded, but with what? In the mind of the people, he was a hero; there was that. Otherwise, his Court rank had been increased from *spatharios* to *protospatharios*, and his Court salary had been only moderately increased. But the lack of prestige and material gain disturbed him much less than the tedious conditions of his job. Had he suffered so much, had he risked his life, merely to investigate cases of petty embezzlement?

He knew he wasn't chasing glory. His present position did not suffice for him because he wanted to do something that mattered, both to himself and to the Empire.

Well, of course he was impractical—impractical enough to have fallen in love with a woman whose parents surely considered him far beneath them. She appeared to have a different opinion although he was not quite certain that she returned his feelings. True, she managed to see him from time to time when she came to the Great Palace with her teacher, the Court Physician. And occasionally he found an excuse to visit the Court Physician's office. But he did not know when he would see her again.

Certainly not today, not the way things were turning out. For the present, he might as well resign himself to routine. One always had that to fall back on.

"I'll probably be home this noon," he said, "to catch up on my sleep."

George grunted in acknowledgement. "See you then. I'll have the boy get off his scrawny butt—excuse me—to thank you."

Michael rode out the gate. As he turned onto a byway dominated by the blank facades of several mansions, a contingent of mounted men clattered towards him. Most of them wore the gold-trimmed red tunics of the Varangian Guard, the Emperor's Russo-Scandinavian bodyguards.

As soon as they caught sight of Michael, they reined in. "Good!" exclaimed the commander of the Varangians, a tall, broad-shouldered Russian with a closely-trimmed blond beard. "We hoped to catch you before you got to the Palace."

"Actually, I was headed in the opposite direction," said Michael. "I was going to the Monastery of the Studion. Today's the feast day of—"

"Sorry, but you'll have to come with us."

"Yes," added Constantine Psellus, the only civilian in the group. "We've sent more men to fetch your superior." A thin, stoop-shouldered man whose dull brown hair and beard were nearly the same color as his clothing, Psellus was the Emperor's First Secretary and head of the Faculty of Philosophy at the state-run university.

Michael's eyes widened. "What's going on? What have I—" He felt a spasm of fear. Not so long ago he had been accused of murder.

"We're putting you on a case," said Psellus. "One of your colleagues in the Post has been strangled."

11

Chapter 4

Yelling "Make way!" to the startled passers-by and shoppers crowding the Mese, Michael and his escort sped their horses westward, up the hill of the Holy Apostles. When they passed the massive five-domed church itself, they slowed their mounts to a walk, and the commander of Varangians—the Akoluthos—rode out in front. "It can't be far now," he said, as they passed through the ruins of the old City wall. "They'll have a man waiting for us."

Just ahead, a militiaman in the roadway waved them down with his club. "Down here!" he gestured to his left. They followed him down the hillside, toward a grove of beech trees. Nearby, several hobbled horses grazed placidly. As Michael and his party dismounted, they could hear the murmur of voices, punctuated by a few desultory barks.

Inside the grove they found three more Varangians, as well as George Blachernites, Michael's superior, the Logothete of the Dromos, head of the Imperial Post. A slight, white-haired man, he dipped his head to acknowledge their arrival, then indicated the others in the group: two militiamen, fingering the clubs hanging at their belts, and the pair of farmers who had discovered the body. They all looked uneasily at a supine form covered with a cloak.

"It's Bourtzes," said Blachernites, knitting his white brows.

Michael crossed himself. "Eustathios Bourtzes?" Indeed, there was only one Bourtzes in the Post, and he was a legend. Back in September, when Constantinople had been besieged by Tornicius's rebels, Bourtzes infiltrated the enemy camp, impersonated a rebel soldier, and obtained vital intelligence. Moreover, the previous winter, he investigated the activities of the Patzinaks, the fierce steppe nomads who had settled in the Empire's western provinces.

"I thought he was out on a mission," said Michael.

"He just came back," said Blachernites. "But he never reached the Great Palace to deliver his report."

Michael scratched the nape of his neck. "How did he—"

"Hell knows how he got here!" the Logothete replied.

"Obviously he was attacked," said the Akoluthos.

One of the militiamen spoke. "He had only a few coppers in his belt pouch, so he could have been robbed. And look at his clothes!" Bourtzes's tunic and hose were torn in several places. Dirt and flakes of dry leaves had been ground into the fine wool.

"He could have been moved—dragged—from somewhere else," the militiaman added.

"And could have put up a fight," said Michael.

The militiaman bent down and reached for the victim's right hand. "But look!"

Michael nodded. "His fingernails are unbroken—and clean!" What? Surely Bourtzes had been a master of self-defense. Had he been taken by surprise?

Michael glanced at the Logothete, who was scowling. Did he have similar thoughts?

"And where is his horse?" Blachernites demanded. "He must have been riding a post horse."

That, Michael thought, was a rhetorical question. Who

could answer it?

"Ah—I'd like to take a look at the body," he said, though he hardly relished the prospect.

One of the militiamen drew back the cloak covering Bourtzes. The farmers exclaimed loudly and crossed themselves, then moved away.

Michael knelt beside the corpse, noting Bourtzes's matted black hair, bluish lips, and blotched facial skin. His eyes, flecked with blood and glazed over, were still open.

"Strangulation, you see," pronounced the militiaman. Michael rose—though not without tangling himself in his long legs—and tasted bile. He covered his mouth with a handkerchief. *Steady! You'll just have to get used to it.*

He wiped his mouth and spoke. "At least the scavengers haven't been at him, thank God. And thanks, no doubt, to our friends the dogs."

The Akoluthos nodded, then knelt down and pulled at Bourtzes's collar. He indicated the narrow red line around Bourtzes's neck. "A thin cord, a bowstring, anything of the sort could have done the job. It doesn't give us much to go on."

For who didn't have rope or string in his house? Michael thought. And not only military archers used a bow. Many civilians used it for hunting, or for protecting their households. He would have to find a means to identify the murderer other than by the weapon he used. But now he didn't even know the essential facts of this case.

"Once again, how was the body found?"

One of the militiamen beckoned the farmers back, while the Akoluthos pulled the cloak over Bourtzes's face.

"We keep cows," began the elder farmer. "And we live down there." He gestured in the direction of the valley. "This morning, when we let them out, the dogs went wild. They ran up here, and—"

"Can your farmstead be seen from here?" Michael asked.

"Yes. I'll show you."

Michael, accompanied by the Akoluthos, Blachernites, and Psellus, followed the farmers out of the grove.

"There," said the graybeard, indicating some stone buildings down the slope.

"So." Michael could not recall seeing another occupied house or farm close by. Back near the ruins of the old City wall, the buildings had thinned out.

"Did you hear or see anything suspicious last night?" he asked.

"The dogs started barking," said the younger farmer.

"At what time was that?"

"I don't know, but it was late. We'd all gone to bed. We told the dogs to shut up, but we weren't afraid because they were inside with us."

"So, they must have sensed some activity up here?"

"I guess they did."

Michael nodded. Sometime during the night, Bourtzes had come here, either alive or dead. That fact wasn't much help, but it was a beginning.

"And this morning they charged up here as soon as you let them out?" Michael eyed them. They were now chasing each other near the grazing cows.

"Yes."

"You'd never seen this man before?"

"No!" chimed both farmers.

Michael thought they were telling the truth. "Well?" he asked, glancing at the Logothete of the Dromos. Was he convinced?

But before Blachernites could answer, a newcomer spoke up. "Your Excellencies?"

They turned. A stocky Varangian Guard addressed them. "The wagon has arrived."

"Good," said Psellus, twisting a strand of his mousy brown beard. "He'll take...Bourtzes back to the Palace. The doctor can examine him, and then he can be prepared for burial."

"Yes. And we'll notify the family," said the Logothete of the Dromos. He paused and drew his white brows together. "But I want his horse found. He should have been carrying important documents."

Chapter 5

The silver early-afternoon sun crept in through the narrow windows of the hall of the Varangian Guard, falling on the thick fair hair of Emperor Constantine Monomachus. The light emphasized the pallor of his swollen features.

He slumped in his heavy chair on the dais, shifting his position only when the pangs of his gout struck him. A semicircle of Varangians stood behind him while the Akoluthos, positioned at a small table to the Emperor's left, rustled parchments and made a few notes.

Facing the dais, Michael and other Court officials occupied the lower portion of the hall. They stood passively, hands at their sides, and waited for the Court physician to arrive. He would tell them what he'd found on Bourtzes's corpse.

The Emperor, rustling his long purple tunic, leaned toward Michael. The pendant jewels on his domed crown swung back and forth. "Thanks to your help in the Tornicius affair, we've decided to put you in charge of this investigation." Inclining his head stiffly, he addressed the Logothete of the Dromos. "That's agreeable to you, isn't it, Your Excellency?"

"Of course."

The Emperor faced Michael again. "So, Taronites, you'll have the support of your department, the Varangians, and our esteemed First Secretary."

A smile flickered across Psellus's thin lips.

Michael bowed his head. "I thank you, Your Majesty."

He looked up and posed his first question. "So, who had any reason to kill him?"

The Emperor tilted his leonine head to one side. "It's hard to believe he had any enemies. He was an honest, upright man, and a good Christian—God rest his soul!"

Psellus snorted. "He waged a personal war against evil. Such people have many enemies—at least in this world."

One or two Varangians laughed, then thought better of it.

"Ahem!" said Blachernites. "I can think of one or two conflicts."

"What?" asked Michael. The Akoluthos poised his pen, while the other courtiers waited.

"Last winter I sent Bourtzes to the Danube frontier, to investigate the Patzinaks who had settled on our side of the river. One of their notables that he spied on was Metiga, nephew of the war leader Kegen, head of all the Patzinaks who found refuge with us. Earlier this same Metiga had come to the City as an ambassador to the Court. He's here now, and he makes his presence known. But I digress…"

The Akoluthos regarded him with stern gray eyes. "Yes, stick to your story."

"Here's what happened. Last winter, around the Feast of the Nativity, Kegen's Patzinaks got themselves mindlessly drunk and stayed so for several days. Most of them are heathens, as you might think, though some few are Christians. Nevertheless, I'm sure that they all use the winter solstice as an excuse for a good debauch; that's one thing they're all agreed on."

"At that time, Metiga went into the nearest town, to

make merry in his own way. But while he was absent, Tirakh Khan, Kegen's rival, brought his own Patzinaks across the Danube ice and attacked Kegen's people, who were in no condition to fight."

Michael could see what was coming.

"The local civil and military officials were up in arms, so Bourtzes undertook an investigation of that incident and questioned Metiga about his whereabouts at the critical time. Did he cross the ice to the north shore of the Danube and invite Tirakh Khan to attack? No, Metiga claimed. He had merely gone to Silistria to patronize the taverns and brothels. He insisted that he had been laid up dead drunk, for two days, in one of the latter establishments, and had no knowledge of the invasion."

"Was his claim proved?"

"Nothing was ever proved against him. Bourtzes questioned the proprietors and employees of those...houses, and they all vouched for Metiga."

"He could very well be innocent," said Michael, "though he might resent Bourtzes for questioning his integrity."

"Yes," said the Logothete, "since inciting a horde of barbarians to make war on Imperial soil is tantamount to treason. And whatever caused Tirakh Khan to bring his men over, we're now living with the results of that disaster."

"What is Metiga's status now?" Michael asked.

"He's still an ambassador of his people," said the Logothete, "though he was never considered very important. But he's lodging at an inn, all his expenses paid by—Your Majesty," he added, glancing at the Emperor. "So, any suspicions against him haven't harmed his position."

Psellus chewed on his moustache. "However, the two Patzinak factions fight each other, and both make war on us."

Michael nodded. He feared the Emperor had made a fatal error of policy in allowing Kegen's people to settle within the Empire. Far from defending the frontier, they had brought more trouble inside it—enough trouble to cause most residents of the western provinces to side with the notorious rebel Tornicius.

Michael spoke. "Who besides Metiga had a possible quarrel with Bourtzes?"

Psellus turned away. "Ah—no one, really."

Michael cocked an eyebrow. "No one?"

The Logothete of the Dromos cleared his throat.

Michael faced him, then Psellus. What were they hiding?

"Oh, it's nonsense—nothing, really," said the Logothete of the Dromos. "It's the matter of the chief of His Majesty's household."

Michael felt a chill creep up his back. He'd sent his servant's son to a man who might be involved in Bourtzes's death.

Blachernites took a step towards the dais. "I wash my hands of the matter."

The Emperor chuckled. "Oh, come now. The Rector is a good fellow. He just likes to have his little joke."

"I see," said Michael, though from what he'd heard, the head of the Imperial household, a former soapmaker, liked his jokes obscene and scatological. And since the Emperor shared his taste, both Psellus and Blachernites were reluctant to criticize him.

"Saponas…" Michael began. "What did Bourtzes have to do with him?"

"Very, little," said the Logothete, "except for the fact that Bourtzes expressed his disapproval to Saponas's face on numerous occasions."

"That hardly constitutes a motive for murder." Michael paused and looked up at the Emperor. "Ah—especially since I gather that Saponas still enjoys Your Majesty's favor."

"He does," said the Emperor, with an expansive wave of his hand.

Thus far, Michael had learned little that was useful. "Who else had a reason to kill Bourtzes?"

Blachernites nudged him and whispered. "You know about Tripsychos?"

Michael's reply was louder. "My colleague in the Post, Gregory Tripsychos."

The Emperor raised his fair eyebrows. "Now, what's this?"

"Oh, it's an old personal rivalry," said the Logothete.

"Over a woman?" The Emperor laughed gracefully.

"At least in part," Blachernites replied.

"Ah!" the Akoluthos broke in. "Remember what happened last spring?"

Blachernites winced. "Of course." He cleared his throat, then spoke: "Both men were waiting to see me. Without thinking about it, I received Bourtzes in my office first; it's what I usually did. But Tripsychos took offense, called Bourtzes a boot-licker, and struck him. 'You get everywhere first,' he said. Bourtzes replied that he'd earned whatever he had, and hit back. Then—"

"Some of my men had to break it up," said the Akoluthos. "Bourtzes and Tripsychos were punching each other all over the hallway, spilling each other on the floor, and using language that would make a Saracen camel-driver blanch."

"Well!" said Michael. "Then I'll need to question Tripsychos as well. It seems we need to interview three men—and learn their whereabouts last night. I presume that's when Bourtzes was killed."

"And we must question the night guards at the City walls," said the Logothete. "We know the postern gate where Bourtzes was expected."

"Where can I find our present suspects?" Michael asked.

"Metiga has rooms at an inn," said the Emperor. "Saponas has quarters here in the Great Palace, but he also owns a house and factory in the soapmakers' district."

"And Tripsychos has a house on the west side, in the Psamathia quarter," said the Logothete. "Most likely you'll find him there. He was wounded last Thursday and has been ill since then."

"Wounded?" asked Michael.

"By brigands," said the Logothete. "He was on an assignment."

At these words, the Emperor straightened himself from his invalid's slump and turned serious. "Taronites, we need to discuss Bourtzes's own assignment: as you may know, he was gone for six weeks. He was incognito, and his purpose was known to only three people besides ourselves: to the Logothete of the Dromos, to the *Kanikleios*—the Custodian of the Imperial Inkstand—and..."

"What about him?" asked Michael.

"He and Bourtzes were barely acquainted," said the Emperor.

"Oh. But you mentioned a third person, Your Majesty. Who was he?"

"Nicetas Saponas, the head of my household. He happened to be in the room at the time."

"How is that possible?" Michael demanded.

Again, Blachernites nudged Michael. "I'll tell you later. And I'll tell you about the mission."

"So." The Akoluthos set down his pen. His gray eyes were expressionless. "What was Bourtzes carrying on his return? Any dispatches?"

"He should have been," said the Logothete of the Dromos. "But as you know, we still haven't found his horse and saddlebags. And there were only a few coins in his belt pouch."

Come now! thought Michael. "You're implying that he was killed for his money?"

Blachernites set his lips. After a moment's silence, he spoke. "That doesn't seem likely, does it? Though the culprit could have used theft as a cover for something else."

"True," said Michael. "However,..." He paused, pursuing an elusive thought. "Did anyone know just when Bourtzes would return?"

"No one knew," said the Emperor," though the guards at the walls were instructed to watch for him as long as necessary."

"No one," Michael repeated, pondering Monomachus's

words.

But now the double doors behind them whooshed open. Michael turned to see them close behind a solitary figure— the Court physician, a tall though paunchy eunuch in a silk robe of physician's blue. All eyes turned toward him as he made his way up the central aisle.

Andronicus Acropolites, the physician was usually a friendly, kindly person, but today his face was set, resembling a painted mask.

Michael was not the only one who noticed. The Logothete of the Dromos drew an impatient, expectant breath as the doctor prostrated himself before the Emperor.

Michael fidgeted with his belt.

"You've examined the body," the Emperor inquired. "Tell us what you found."

Acropolites ascended the dais and turned to face the courtiers. Though his smooth, fair-skinned face gave nothing away, he clenched his hands across his stomach. For a long moment he regarded the group in silence, then coughed and spoke in a ringing contralto. "As previously determined, the victim died of strangulation by a very common type of ligature. But...well..." He swallowed hard. "He was also raped."

Chapter 6

"**H**e was *what?*" demanded Michael. The Emperor set his slips and suppressed a groan. The courtiers shuffle their feet and muttered either prayers or curses. Psellus's mouth worked, as though he were choking back bile.

The eyes of the Akoluthos met the physician's. "Are you certain?"

"There is every indication," said Acropolites. "However, despite the...trauma, there was no blood loss to speak of."

"That will do!" said Blachernites.

"Excuse me," said the doctor, and continued. "So, we can conclude that Bourtzes was already dead."

The Akoluthos broke his pen in two and tossed it away. "Well, that's a mercy!"

"God rest his soul," someone exclaimed. The others in the room mumbled their assent, crossing themselves hastily.

The back of Michael's neck prickled. Like the others, he warded off an evil that has come much too close.

The Emperor, raising a bloated hand, signaled to Psellus. The latter promptly ascended the dais, wiped the Imperial brow with a handkerchief of purple silk, and helped his master find a more comfortable position.

Now color surged into the Emperor's cheeks. "What monster has done this?" he demanded, his words reverberating against the vaulted ceiling.

Michael bowed his head in thought. The question, of course, was purely rhetorical.

§

The Emperor, who had neither the strength nor the stomach to continue the inquiry, dismissed his officials almost immediately. Michael approached Acropolites on the way out. "Come over to my office," said the physician.

Michael thought of Olympia Macrembolitissa, the physician's student, and felt himself blush; Acropolites enjoyed throwing Michael and the young lady together. "Er—I'll come as soon as possible, but first I need to report to my superior."

They parted, and Michael headed deep into the Palace compound. He struck off across an open courtyard, then downhill towards the octagonal gold-domed Chrysotriclinium, the most sumptuous throne room. The offices of the Post were in a wing built onto the back.

The Logothete's door was open, and Michael found the lithe little man bent over his desk, his face in his hands. At the sound of Michael's footsteps, he scraped his chair back on the marble floor and stood up.

"Well, have a seat." He indicated an austere-looking armchair on one of several Persian carpets.

"Thank you, sir." Michael sank onto the thinnish cushion.

"May I get you a drink?" The Logothete crossed to a cabinet on the far side of the room and poured wine from a silver ewer into two goblets. "Water?" he asked.

"No thank you." Then Michael jumped to his feet. "Sir, I should be waiting upon you."

"Never mind." Blachernites reached for the ewer again, the filled both cups to the brim. "This occasion calls for something strong."

Michael nodded, and sank back into his chair. The room was warmed heated by two braziers burning charcoal and aromatic wood. But still he shivered.

He gratefully accepted the wine and, to his own surprise, downed half the cup at one gulp. Its heavy sweetness warmed his stomach and seeped into his limbs. "Can you tell me now just what Bourtzes was doing in the provinces. I gather you didn't want to mention it in front of everyone."

Blachernites sank into his own chair. "It will be common knowledge soon enough, once this investigation gets underway. At this point secrecy no longer matters. Bourtzes is dead; someone else may have the information we need, and unless we recover Bourtzes's dispatches, we won't learn what we need to."

"Which is—"

"I sent him to investigate sedition of a certain kind."

Michael startled. "Sedition? But almost all Tornicius's followers abandoned him after his siege failed, after His Majesty promised them amnesty."

"I'm speaking of a different sort of rebels. Bourtzes went to Philippopolis."

"Ah! You mean he was investigating heretics? Manicheans? What is the sect back there called— Bogomils?"

"You're right. But actually, there's quite a selection of sects back there." A scowl crossed the Logothete's face. "Of course, now we're mainly concerned with the Bogomil faith, the latest version of the old Manichean or dualist error. It's spread like wildfire among the Slav population."

Michael narrowed his eyes. "I can see why we need to be concerned: they preach sedition."

"Indeed. They say that governments, like everything else visible or material, are the work of the devil."

"They're potentially disloyal," said Michael, "but have they actually committed a treasonous act?"

"That's what we want to find out. We know from experience that these sects can assume an aggressive role. Take the Paulicians, whose beliefs are similar to the Bogomils'. They find it expedient to make war on the 'wicked' authorities."

Michael rested his goblet on his knee. "But the Empire defeated them long ago."

"The sect still exists. The authorities resettled many of their number at Philippopolis."

"So Bourtzes was to spy on them also?" Michael sipped his wine pensively.

"Yes." Blachernites got up and began to pace the floor. "Now—back to the Bogomils. Unlike the Paulicians, they eschew warfare. They resist authority passively, refusing to obey what they call the laws of the devil. Or so they say."

Michael raised an eyebrow. "You mean that in practice, they might find some justification for war?"

"Exactly. They've been known to put on a mask for the outside world. On the other hand, if they truly adhere to their pacifism, they might allow another group to fight for them."

"Ah," said Michael. "I can see possibilities there. And so Bourtzes was sent to Philippopolis to discover just how much damage they've done."

28

"Yes." The Logothete sat down again. He drained his cup and eyed the ewer on the cabinet but thought better of taking another drink. "However, that's no easy task, thanks to the Bogomils' deceitfulness. They're skilled at blending into their surroundings. They often attend Church services and pretend to be Orthodox, and they play the part of exemplary, law-abiding citizens. To them, such behavior isn't hypocritical: they're fooling the devil and his servants."

"Evidently Bourtzes knew more than was good for...someone." Michael's fingers tightened around the stem of his cup.

He was also raped. Once more, the horror of the doctor's words swept over Michael. His stomach pitched, and he gulped the rest of his wine to stem the tide of nausea.

He'd been put in charge of Bourtzes's case, but what did he know of the mystery of evil? He needed the advice of someone older and more experienced. "Did Bourtzes's killer...prefer men?"

At first the Logothete seemed not to hear. He padded across the carpet and refilled his cup, then extended the ewer to Michael.

"No thank you." Determined to keep his wits about him, he set his goblet on the rug.

"As for your concern—not necessarily. Think: why does anyone rape a woman?"

Michael recoiled in shock. What a question! "I don't know. I've never even...thought about it."

Blachernites appeared to regret the wording of his question. "Well, of course you wouldn't. And consider: it's usually an act of scorn, of hatred, or a display of brute force.

That's why it happens so often in wartime…and yes, even to men. Lust is only a secondary impetus."

"That sounds reasonable."

"So, the killer need not have been…of that disposition." The Logothete paused and nodded briskly, recalling something else. "Of course, he could have been a Bogomil. You know the stories people tell about them."

"I don't, really, but what monster would violate a dead man?"

In silence, the Logothete returned to his desk and sat. "A rare one, surely," he said. "But whoever did it also found reason to rob Bourtzes. Remember—we found only a few coppers on him."

Michael wondered why Blachernites was concentrating on this dubious explanation. "They lurked at the streetside and set upon him by chance, then dragged him off the road, killing and robbing him. And they left his body in the beech grove… Now, that's certainly a possibility. That explanation appears to account for everything."

"Appears to?" The Logothete raised his white brows.

"In truth it provokes another question: Bourtzes was skilled in self-defense. How did his assailants overpower him?"

Blachernites winced. "You think there were more than one?"

"Yes, in any case. And it's true—if Bourtzes were killed for political reasons, by conspirators, that leaves much unexplained. Who knew when he was due back from the provinces?"

"Why—you heard what the Emperor said. Nobody

knew—not even myself!"

"That's the difficulty." *At least you say you didn't know!* Michael thought.

"Bourtzes left town a little more than six weeks ago, so it was reasonable to expect him back fairly soon. It might have taken him a week or two to make the two-hundred-and-fifty-mile journey to Philippopolis, since he took a loaded pack mule with him. He'd disguised himself as a government official selling off surplus garments from the Imperial silk workshops. But he could have made the trip back very quickly—in three days, if he'd discovered something important. He had authorization to order a change of horses at each stage along the highway."

Michael sighed. "But did he discover something, or did he seek in vain, and then take his time coming home?"

"I don't know."

Michael leaned forward. "We need to send someone to question officials at the postal stations along his route."

"Ahem. Of course. We'll do it."

"But that will take time. So, let's take a different approach. Once again, let's consider who knew about his mission."

"Besides myself, only the Emperor, Syropoulos, Custodian of the Imperial Inkstand, and, by chance, Nicetas Saponas?"

Saponas? Michael sat up straight. "That's what I wondered about. The head of the Imperial household had no business at a high-security meeting."

Blachernites swore under his breath. "That's what I wanted to tell you, back in the Varangians' hall. Of course, he has not such business, but that buffoon goes wherever he pleases. The Emperor is completely enamored with him—I can think of no other word—and of his vulgar jokes and capacity for drink."

"You're not implying that there's anything...unusual in their relationship?"

The Logothete waved his hand dismissively. "Oh no! It's quite obvious that the Emperor likes only women."

Michael had to agree to that. Currently, the Emperor had an elderly wife and a young mistress.

"Saponas is just another of His Majesty's intense but undiscriminating friendships. Of course, the fool has one good quality. Five years, when Michael the Caulker seized the throne, Saponas joined the popular movement to overthrow the wretch and led a gang of soapmakers in a march on the Palace."

"And that's what's endeared him to our present government."

"Yes."

"But Bourtzes didn't hesitate to express disapproval of Saponas's behavior?"

"On more than one occasion he called the man a coarse buffoon—to his face!"

Michael nodded. "So, there must have been bad feeling between them, though hardly enough for murder. Saponas must have known that Bourtzes's judgment meant little to the Emperor."

"I take your meaning."

"And I think we can rule out the Emperor as a suspect. He authorized the investigation, and it's certainly in his interest to keep the Empire at peace."

"Of course!"

"Now, about Syropoulos," Michael continued. "Did he have any quarrel with Bourtzes?"

"Not that I'm aware of."

"Hm! What about Bourtzes himself. Is there any chance that he was not so upright as he appeared?"

The Logothete sat up, jerking his head back. "Why no! That's never occurred to me. He's the victim here!"

"Yes, of course."

Blachernites went limp; his outburst seemed to have sapped his strength. "We do try to keep track of our agents' private lives, without being intrusive. And while our methods are far from infallible," he added, scowling, "they can turn up a great deal. So, as far as we know, Bourtzes had no extra-marital affairs of any sort. And he didn't get drunk, gamble, or go to brothels."

"So, the man and his legend are one. Still, I wonder about Psellus's remark."

"That good people have enemies? I think he was implying that Bourtzes was somewhat of a prig. Perhaps he was."

As is Psellus, thought Michael. "But though such people are annoying, one doesn't murder them."

"No."

"Now, what about, Metiga, the Patzinak, the one person known to have been on bad terms with Bourtzes?" Could he have known about this mission?"

"Not unless someone told him, and no one had any right to do so."

Michael raised an eyebrow. "Well! But if someone did?"

Blachernites scowled again, no doubt thinking of those present at the meeting. And now Michael recalled just who had been there.

"I must go, if I may," said Michael. He rose from his seat but delivered a parting shot. "The Patzinak's involvement seems absurd, but I'd like to talk to the man. Where can I find him?"

"He's staying at an inn called The Golden Fleece. It's out past the Holy Apostles, near the old Wall of Constantine... And by the way, he has company now—a half-brother, whom he presented at Court last week."

"I'll call on them later," said Michael. "But first I'm going to the Monastery of the Studion. I was on my way there this morning when the Varangians caught up with me. At least I can give my regards to Father Zosimas. I haven't seen him since I came back to town."

"Zosimas?" Knitting his brows, the Logothete rose slowly. "You know him?"

"Yes. He's an old family friend and my spiritual father. Actually, he's the closest thing I have to a father."

"I see. I didn't realize that. Well, good day."

"Good day to you, sir." Michael started for the door. "I'll keep in touch."

But only silence greeted him.

Outside the office, Michael paused. He was puzzled by his superior's reticence about Zosimas, but now he realized that he had felt uneasy all through the interview. All in all, Blachernites had been reticent about the case. Did he know more than he cared to reveal? And why?

Please, let me be mistaken! Michael prayed.

For besides the Emperor, Syropoulos and Saponas, only one other person knew the details of Bourtzes's journey: The Logothete of the Dromos himself.

Chapter 7

Somewhere, a gong rang out the ninth hour. The sun, covered by a veil of cloud, was well on its downward course when Michael arrived at the Monastery of the Studion, in the southwest corner of the City. Once he'd been admitted by the porter, he bypassed the timber-roofed, basilical church and headed down a dirt path flanked by cypress trees and the squarish, whitewashed buildings housing the monastery's many workshops. One such structure contained several writing and copying rooms, and it was there that Father Zosimas usually spent the afternoons.

Once inside, Michael paused outside the only open door and peered in. A monk stood at a desk, his long, graying fair hair tucked into the neckline of his habit. His compact, well-formed body bent over some work, and though he could not have been exerting himself, he appeared to be struggling under a great weight. It was Zosimas, and he was alone.

Michael wondered why the monk had come here at all today. On the feast-day of St. Theodore the Studite, a one-time abbot of the monastery who had fearlessly defended the holy icons before emperors and false bishops, surely Zosimas would not be engaged in any serious labors.

Michael took a tentative step into the room. "Father?"

Zosimas dropped his pen and spun around with the agility of a young man. His dark, threadbare garment gave off a pungent scent of incense. He breathed deeply, and his blue eyes, surrounded by fine wrinkles, widened.

"Michael! *Chaire!* Rejoice," he said, using the ancient

greeting. "I didn't think you'd returned yet."

"I'm sorry I startled you." Michael approached to kiss his hand. "I came back last night. I was planning to come to the service this morning, but I was called out on an emergency. One of my colleagues was murdered."

Zosimas crossed himself. "God rest his soul. Who was it?"

"Eutstathios Bourtzes. That's a pity, isn't it?"

"Yes. From what I've heard, he was a good man. If we had more such—"

"He wasn't only murdered. He was also raped."

The monk sucked in his breath and crossed himself again. He squeezed his eyes shut.

Michael shrank. "I'm sorry but talking about it helps."

Zosimas opened his eyes and looked up at Michael. "Of course. I understand." He indicated a stool. "Come sit down," he said and sank onto another.

Michael sat awkwardly. His legs were too long. "So, what are you doing here today?"

"Just cleaning up." Zosimas indicated a stack of parchment scraps, a penknife and pens, and a pile of shavings on the desk behind him.

"I mean—what are you working on now?"

The monk's smile was half-hidden in his beard. "I'm between projects now, or just cleaning up after the last one."

"You are?" Michael was surprised that he did not say more.

"Well, how was your trip?"

"It was a routine case. We learned that some postal

officials had been availing themselves of State horses and carriages for their personal use."

"Oh." There was a hint of amusement in Zosimas's eyes, but it quickly vanished. "Is something else troubling you?"

Michael let his shoulders slump. "I know I should be grateful. I came so close to being convicted of murder. But somehow everything is not as I thought it would be."

The monk's shrug was barely visible. "Really?"

"Though His Majesty gave me a higher rank and transferred me to the Post, he's done nothing to increase my Court salary—not that I really care about that."

"I understand." Zosimas looked up at him. "This Emperor is not known for keeping his promises. Still, the authorities must have confidence in you if they've put you in charge of such a...sensitive case."

Michael straightened himself. "I suppose you're right."

But a door creaked somewhere in the building, and Michael lost his train of thought. Soft footfalls approached the room, then stopped short.

"Who's that?" asked Michael.

"I don't know. I'd pay no attention." A smile flashed across the monk's face. "Now, as you were saying..."

"I understand my good fortune, but I'm still dissatisfied."

"Listen, it's a good thing for a virtuous man to make his way in the world and influence others for good. But one should never forget that the world itself lies in wickedness. That's one reason there are so many of us in here." Zosimas indicated the whole monastery complex with a sweep of his hand. "Of course, we should all be here for other reasons,

38

not simply that the world is so bad."

Michael cocked an eyebrow. "You're right, the world hasn't improved much, not even after we put down that rebellion."

Zosimas threw up his hands. "And alas, it can't improve, so long as people continue to behave dishonorably. Remember everything that's happened recently."

"How could I forget? But what do you mean, specifically?"

"When Tornicius took possession of the western provinces, he made all his officers swear the most fearful oaths of loyalty, oaths sworn on holy relics. Even that wouldn't have been so bad. But when Tornicius was defeated, they forsook him without a qualm. I'm sorry to say that my brother was among them, even though my brother is a decent man, whereas Tornicius is not."

Zosimas's brother was *hypostrategos*—lieutenant-general—of the army of the Theme of Macedonia, and by virtue of this office, also vice-governor of the province. His family, though of Slavonic descent, had long been important in the military hierarchy of the region and owned extensive property near the city of Philippopolis.

"I understand that it grieves you," said Michael.

"But 'our side' is no better," continued Zosimas. "Monomachus promised amnesty to Tornicius, also swearing the most fearful oaths, but he weakened and heeded the evil counsel of certain hard-hearted individuals. He ordered Tornicius blinded, along with the one man who remained loyal to him."

Michael winced. "Yes, that was a wicked deed, but

nobody cares what people of our sort think."

Zosimas was staring at the ceiling. "Of course, Tornicius was hardly above reproach. Though he'd put on the habit of a monk, he took up the sword again."

"As I recall, Tornicius was forcibly tonsured in the first place," said Michael. "That's how Monomachus hoped to bar him from public life. But that was like stuffing a wild boar into a monk's habit—oh, sorry, Father."

Once again, Zosimas smiled his faint, beautiful smile. "Well, you're right about that. And I haven't even mentioned our greatest shame: the tax-collectors who wring exorbitant sums from poor farmers and force them to sell out to landlords who rob them all over again."

"Our publicans are no better than cannibals."

"It's true—I know. I'm not so naïve—especially not since…well, that's not important." Zosimas broke off, as though his words were choking him. "Ahem—as I was saying, the world is wicked, but there are some brave souls who can persevere in it untainted. I think you're one of them," he added, clapping a hand on Michael's shoulder. "For others, the only wise course of action is to enter a monastery."

"Yes, everyone should examine himself," said Michael, hoping he didn't sound pompous.

"You know, lately I've often thought that your father should have been a monk. Poor Theodore!" He crossed himself.

A pain clenched Michael's vitals, as always when he thought of his father's death. "In that case, I wouldn't be here—but yes."

"I didn't mean it that way," said Zosimas. "Your father was always an honorable, upright soul, and he couldn't comprehend that most people are just the opposite." Zosimas had known Michael's father since his youth, when they were both students at Constantinople's School of the Holy Apostles.

Michael took a rasping breath. "In the end he learned just how evil people could be—when his enemies tried to ruin him, when they concocted those absurd charges of attempting to murder the Caulker." He struggled to keep his voice even. "Oh, I know he took the betrayal too hard, even after the Empress Zoe cleared him. What else could have driven him to drink?"

"Still, he had more virtues than weaknesses," said Zosimas. "But they might have been put to better use in a monastery. Whereas I, on the other hand... Perhaps I should have been a soldier, like my brother and my forefathers. Certainly, it's easier to face an evil you can fight against."

"A soldier, you?" Yet the idea was not utterly preposterous: Zosimas came from good, healthy stock.

"Oh, I know that's ridiculous. But such are the vain thoughts of an old man."

"You're not old."

"Sometimes I feel ancient." Zosimas folded his hands in his lap. "However—" He broke off and looked towards the door.

Michael followed his gaze and saw a dark-clad form skitter past. "Who was that?"

"I don't know."

Outside, the sun emerged from behind the clouds. Bright, orange light spilled in through the bare windows, emphasizing the lines on Zosimas's face and the white hairs in his beard. Though the room seemed warmer, Michael shivered involuntarily.

For a moment, Zosimas watched him in silence, then spoke. "Let's talk about you now, and the lady doctor. Have you…"

"Technically, she's still a student. And nothing has really changed. I see her only occasionally, at the physician's office. Sometimes I'm certain that she's…interested, and at other times, I'm not certain at all."

"Of course, I know nothing of such matters," Zosimas replied, smiling. "But sometimes young women—especially intelligent women—are reluctant to enter into marriage. They might prefer to embrace the monastic life, or they might be reluctant to lose their autonomy, or their accomplishments."

"What autonomy, when their fathers are constantly looking over their shoulders?"

"That's true enough. But a possibility—a hope—remains."

"And Lady Olympia's father would surely disapprove of me. Of course, if I had more money, a decent house, and powerful relatives, he'd think differently.'"

"Come now! Your father was known as an honorable man, and you're still considered a hero. Our people are not that fickle."

Michael snorted. "One can't live on honor—or on heroics."

"'Man does not live by bread alone.'"

Michael startled. Zosimas was usually not so blunt in his preaching.

Zosimas smiled again. "If I don't say that, who will? And our people—especially the wealthy, tend to forget that consent and mutual love are essential to a marriage. They concentrate on the business aspects."

"That's true."

"I'll pray for you both," said Zosimas. "If it's God's will..."

Michael bowed his head. "I thank you." For the first time today, he felt at peace. Zosimas's unwavering, unhypocritical affection enveloped him like a blanket.

They rose from their seats but remained silent until, outside, the clanging of a metal gong rent the air.

"It's time for Vespers," said Zosimas. "I didn't realize it was so late."

"I can't stay. There are things I must attend to."

§

By the time Michael reached the north side of the Lycus valley, light had bled from the sky. Only a thin zone of gold remained on the western horizon. It was growing colder, and Michael shivered and huddled his beard into his wool cloak. If he intended to examine anything, he had better hurry.

He urged his horse up the long slope leading to the Mese and gazed to his right, towards the heavily populated area of the City. He was not far from the place Bourtzes's corpse had been found.

Yes, here were several stone buildings, already swathed

in shadows. They belonged to the farmers who had discovered the body. And further off lay the beech grove, a dark blotch on the gray, colorless grass of the pasture.

He was perhaps fifty feet below the roadway when more trees and a stone barn, its roof beams exposed, loomed before him. He hadn't noticed it on his previous visit in the area.

He rode closer and peered into the gaping hole of the doorway. "Hello? Is anybody there?"

An echo replied.

Acting on instinct, he looked around warily. Abandoned or not, this place gave him the shivers. He'd come back some other time—in broad daylight. Now he'd concentrate on his other task: to find Metiga the Patzinak.

He reached the Mese and road east, towards the five domes of the Holy Apostles, limned in the distance against the darkening sky.

Around him, the main street wended its way through fields and farm plots. Houses were few and often far from the roadway. Yes, it was a good place for murder. Only when he reached the occasional mansions and the clusters of smaller houses near the old city wall did he rein in. Here glowing windows and street lamps cast a reassuring light on the paving stones. The domestic clatter of pots and pans comforted him.

A militiaman stood just ahead, beside the tumbledown Wall of Constantine.

"Which way to the Golden Fleece?" asked Michael.

"On your right."

Michael followed the man's directions. There, set back a

good twenty-five feet from a side street, rose a three-storied building with carved double doors set into its stuccoed façade. It towered over the neighboring houses, though not over the trees behind it.

Impressive! Michael thought, as he pulled the bell chain and waited for someone to answer.

"I have an appointment with the proprietor," he fibbed, when a pair of servants answered the door. "Can you take care of my horse?" He extracted a pair of silver coins from his belt pouch and pressed them into their hands.

"Your beast'll be out back sir. Go on in."

Once Michael was inside, another servant closed the doors behind him as he surveyed the spacious anteroom. Oil lamps burned overhead in a brass chandelier, and the tessellated floor appeared freshly swept. A broad wooden staircase rose to the second story. Faint but pleasant odors of wine, hot olive oil, fresh fish, and roasted meat wafted in from the kitchen, making Michael aware of the hollow in his stomach.

Yes, this establishment was more than decent: it was luxurious.

But, at the moment, the young man who sat at a large desk commanded his attention.

"I'm looking for Metiga the Patzinak and his brother."

The clerk looked up. "I'm afraid you've missed them."

Michael bit his lip. "They haven't checked out, have they?"

"Oh no. They're just out for the night—as usual. Come around noon tomorrow." He waved his hand expansively. "Then they usually order a meal sent up. They might even be disposed to receive guests."

Michael drew a parchment from his pocket and thrust it under the clerk's nose, making certain that the man also got a look at his signet ring. "I'm from the Post, and I have some questions to ask them. Since they're not here, I'd like to search their rooms."

The clerk's eyes widened. "Oh dear. Oh dear!" He jumped to his feet. "I'd better call the proprietor... Sir? Sir?" He bustled off, returning moments later with a burly, florid-faced man wearing a long tunic of dark wool. The keys on an iron ring at his belt rattled loudly as he walked. "Er— may I help you?" The clatter increased as he bowed.

"I'm Michael Taronites, an agent of the Post."

Color drained from the innkeeper's face. "The—ah— Post?"

"You may be aware that one of our people was found strangled this morning, not far from here."

The proprietor shrank. "Yes, I heard something about it. But I don't know—"

"I'm sure you don't," said Michael, adopting a reassuring tone. He had been on the wrong side of authority himself and saw no point in frightening the man needlessly. "But we think that Metiga, your guest, might have some useful information."

"At night he and his brother go *out*."

"So your clerk says. Where?"

"Oh, drinking and carousing."

The clerk guffawed.

"Ask after them at any of the taverns in the area," said the proprietor. "They'll point them out to you."

"What time do you expect them back?"

"I don't keep track of their comings and goings. Metiga is a privileged guest and has a key to the back door."

Michael raised an eyebrow. "I see. So, they can come in any time they please."

"Yes."

"What about last night? Do you have any idea when they came back?" Michael looked from the proprietor to the clerk."

"No," said the proprietor.

Neither man was much help. "I repeat," said Michael. "I'd like to search their rooms."

The proprietor bowed again, his keys clinking. "Anything you say, Your Honor."

Then, with a stout candlestick in hand, he led Michael to the second floor. He fit a huge iron key into a frontward-facing door to the left of the stairs, then went in and lit the lamps.

The golden light revealed a spacious sitting room with a worn Persian carpet on the floor. The chamber itself looked freshly swept, though it stank of sweat and horses, the scent of its occupants. A round table, several chairs, piles of silk cushions, and a brazier—now cold—were the only furnishings.

Two sets of saddlebags had been tossed into a corner, as well as a large, bulbous wineskin. Michael surmised that this did not contain wine, but *koumis,* a potation of fermented mare's milk that the Patzinaks drank.

"So," began Michael, "Metiga has company."

"Yes, his half-brother came to visit him. I had another

bed brought in." The proprietor gestured towards an inner door.

"Has he been here long?"

"About a week."

"Has Metiga altered his routine in any way since his brother's arrival?"

"No. He comes and goes as he pleases. They both come and go."

"I see." What had Michael expected? He eyed the bedroom door, eager to begin his search.

Sensing Michael's impatience, the proprietor spoke. "Your Honor, you're free to look around. I'll leave you the key." He bowed deeply, then removed it from the ring, and, with a clatter, dropped it on the table. Then, picking up a small bronze lamp, he entered the bedroom.

It stank! More sweat and horses!

Once he'd grown used to the reek, he began to examine his surroundings. Even in the feeble lamplight he could distinguish two wooden beds with rumpled coverlets. Framed by a curtained window, a table with a basin, pitcher, ever, and two cups stood between the beds. Next to each, on the floor, lay two sturdy recurved bows, one stored in its case, one free and ready to be strung.

But Michael had already decided not to concentrate on the bowstring as a possible murder weapon. It was a common object, no more sinister than a table knife.

On the other hand, if he found Bourtzes's missing dispatches—

Grumbling, he looked under the beds, then shook out the bedding, then turned his attention to a pile of clothing flung over a chair. The garment on top was a long garment of green silk brocade.

Michael set down the lamp and picked it up. Its skirt was split in both front and back, to facilitate riding. Very handsome—though definitely in the barbarian style. Up on the steppes, a similar piece of clothing would be made of smelly hides.

Michael found nothing in it and searched the rest of the clothes: loose linen shirts and breeches of cloth or animal skin.

Nothing! Exhaling in exasperation, he piled the garments back on the chair and returned to the sitting room.

Here a look under the rug also proved fruitless, and he proceeded to examine the cushions, pinching and pounding them all. He succeeded only in raising dust.

At this point the wineskin caught his eye. He sniffed the contents and shook it. Indeed, it contained only the nomads' foul brew. Last of all, he went through the saddlebags, which contained only some rather grimy drawers, felt hats, wonder of wonders—a comb—and some extra bowstrings.

Again—nothing important. He extinguished the lamps and locked the door behind him. His next stop would be the stables.

There, the groom was dozing at the door, a lantern beside him.

"Excuse me, I'm from the Post."

The groom rubbed his eyes, then jumped to attention. "Yes, sir."

"I've come for my horse, but first I need to ask some questions and have a look around."

"Of course, sir."

"Never mind. Let's just go in."

The groom picked up the lantern and ushered Michael into a shadowy, low-ceilinged place redolent of dung and hay. It was a stable like any other, with saddles, tack, ropes, blankets, and buckets arranged on racks or hung on pegs.

"Where are the horses of the Patzinak lords?"

"Down here, sir."

At the far end, then. Michael set out in that direction, the groom at his side. "Were they taken out last night?"

"No."

"Are they usually?"

"No."

The groom paused at the third stall to the end. "Here, sir. Lord Metiga brought two horses with him, but his kinsman rode in with only one."

Michael examined them. Their sleek tails swished from side to side. Their coats glistened. They were smaller than the horses of the Empire, and certainly faster. And the Patzinaks themselves, like the steppe nomads of earlier ages, possessed a legendary skill and speed on horseback. What couldn't they do while riding? It was no wonder that in ages past, some benighted souls had believed the mounted tribes to be centaurs—half horse and half man.

"Fine horses," said Michael.

The groom slipped into a stall and patted its occupant on the mane. "There now, boy! It's all right." He turned to Michael. "This is one of Metiga's."

Michael stepped into the stall, and stirred up the straw with his foot. He then examined the cracks between the

50

planks of the partitions.

Nothing was hidden there, or in the other two stalls. "Fetch my horse now, please," he told the groom and rode out soon afterwards. He'd head home now. Tonight, the very thought of seeking the Patzinaks worried him.

The sky was dark and clear and pinpointed with stars. A chill north wind blew, and Michael pulled his cloak tight around him. Last night, when Bourtzes died, the weather had been much the same.

An unpleasant thought! Michael clenched the reins in his left hand. His right hand tightened around the hilt of the dagger he now almost always wore. But he still felt far from safe.

Once he reached the Mese, he urged his horse into a gallop, slowing only when he passed the Holy Apostles. Even then he watched the shadows as he followed the street's lamplit course. He was anxious, but not only because a vicious murderer was on the loose. Fears and doubts had been nagging at him all afternoon.

Why was Blachernites so eager to blame Bourtzes's death on a hypothetical robber, or on the Bogomil sect? Why had he behaved strangely when Michael mentioned Father Zosimas? And what was ailing the monk? What was the evil he had to contend with?

Michael had no answers. And by the time he reached his street, he was too exhausted to think. Fatigue burned his eyes; chills racked his back; an empty ache twisted his stomach. What he needed was a decent meal and some time in the hot room of the public baths. But it was too late for that. And he was not about to order Theodosia, his housekeeper, to prepare anything for him.

But what about a cup of warmed wine or hot water in a basin? Such things were within reason.

But as Michael turned into his unlocked gate, his eyes came wide open. A lantern blazed outside, the stable door, and four arch-necked Arabian horses were tied at the post.

Chapter 8

Clutching his dagger, Michael slid out of the saddle. "Who's there?" he called.

The back door creaked open, and light poured out around a lanky form. "Ah, so there you are!" The voice had a pompous undertone that Michael immediately recognized. It belonged to Constantine Psellus, the Emperor's First Secretary.

Michael sheathed his dagger and raised his hand in acknowledgement. He allowed himself to hope that Psellus had brought good news.

When Michael finally came into the house, Psellus stepped aside. "We hated to disturb you so late, but there have been significant developments. So, we're imposing on your good housekeeper."

"'We?'"

"I brought the Logothete of the Dromos and a pair of guards along. We've taken over your dining room."

Indeed, there all the glass lamps in the hoop chandelier burned brightly. Beneath them, around a table supplied with a wine crock, cups, and a pitcher of water, sat the wiry George Blachernites and two Varangians. Michael's housekeeper stood near the windows, her arms folded across her plump midriff.

Psellus took his seat. Michael bowed to the Logothete, then took his own. He addressed the housekeeper. "Theodosia, could you bring us some more wine and hot water? And you, gentlemen, would you like something to eat?"

"No thank you," chorused Psellus and Blachernites although the Varangians did not decline.

"Well then, please bring us something anyway."

But it was not Theodosia, but Stephen, her son, who returned shortly afterwards, carrying a newly-opened jar of wine. He was a slender young man with a thick, dark beard.

He set the wine on the table and bowed low to Michael. "Thank you for your letter, Your Honor."

"You're quite welcome. Tell me, have you spoken with the Rector yet?"

"He was very kind. He assigned me to his chief groundskeeper," Stephen replied.

"Excellent!" said Michael. His principal concern was that Stephen was employed. And this morning, when Michael had written his letter of recommendation, he had not known that Saponas was a possible suspect for Bourtzes's murder. So if the Rector were dangerous, it was fortunate that Stephen would have no close contact with him.

"So, what will you be doing?" asked Michael.

"Repairs and maintenance, and some gardening during the season."

"Good! Just give it your best."

"Now, Stephen!" His mother returned, carrying a tray with clean cups and a pitcher of hot water. "Run along to bed—if you're going to get up in time."

"Oh, mother!" Stephen thanked Michael once more, then excused himself. Theodosia followed him out.

After everyone had poured themselves wine, Blachernites turned to Michael. "Were you at the monastery all this time?"

"No. I also went to Metiga's inn, but he and his brother were out—as usual, I gather."

"Ha!" broke in Ingvar, the taller and blonder of the Varangians. "I often see Metiga at certain pothouses. Just a few nights ago, he was with another savage."

"*Savage?*" demanded Michael. "You mean his brother, who has recently joined him. Which taverns does he frequent?"

Ingvar recited a whole list, during which the Logothete of the Dromos cleared his throat impatiently.

Afterwards, Michael finished his story. "I searched their rooms and the stables, but in vain."

Psellus creased his brow. "You still plan to question them directly, don't you?"

"Of course—when I catch up with him."

Now Theodosia returned with a plate piled high with sliced, sand-colored bread, a dish of olive oil seasoned with oregano, and a bowl of chick peas soaked in water.

Michael thanked her, and waited till she left the room to pose his next question. "Why are you here?" he asked Blachernites. "What's happened?"

"We've recovered Bourtzes's horse and saddlebags." He knit his white, bushy brows.

Michael poured warm water into his wine. "Since you don't look pleased, I assume they were empty."

"It's not so simple as that."

Michael trembled inwardly. Should he distrust the Logothete? He took a sip and raised one eyebrow. "Indeed not?"

It was Ingvar, not the Logothete who spoke. "This afternoon, a horse with the Post's brand was found running loose on the north side of the City, in the park across from Blachernae Palace. We were notified and came to get it."

"The saddlebags hadn't been stolen," added Blachernites. "They were full of routine letters for Palace officials."

"But no dispatch," said Michael. "Nothing in Bourtzes's hand, with his seal and signature on it?"

"Exactly," said the Logothete. "Nothing addressed to me, or to His Majesty."

Psellus chewed on his mustaches for a moment, then addressed his colleague. "So, what do you think happened?"

Michael wondered if Psellus also distrusted the Logothete. Setting down his cup with a resounding clunk, he made up his mind to speak. "We mean—did the killers take the dispatch, or did Bourtzes plan to make an oral report? Is that customary?"

"No. Because if nothing is recorded, the news could die with its bearer. Still, there are times when it might be expedient to commit nothing to writing, in order to keep information out of the wrong hands. So..." He threw up his hands. "We know nothing! We don't even know if the murderers know what they're looking for."

Psellus swore under his breath. "Oh, if only we knew!"

"We're assuming that there's more than one of them," said Blachernites, "or a murderer and an accomplice. One Bourtzes could have fought."

Michael nodded in agreement. Perhaps the Logothete was truly innocent.

"We must find that dispatch," said Psellus.

"Your Excellency," Ingvar put in, "it's not likely that they just dropped it down a privy."

Michael fingered his cup. "But they've probably destroyed it by now."

"Unfortunately," said Psellus. "But this we do know. We questioned the guards at the postern where Bourtzes entered the City. They say that Bourtzes came through during the second watch of the night. He was headed directly to the Great Palace and said he had some dispatches."

The Logothete nodded. "So! Either he had them then, or he planned to commit his news to writing once he was safe."

"But there's more," continued Psellus. "The guards made one curious observation. When they asked Bourtzes why he'd come in so late, he replied, 'I have my reasons.'"

"Hah! Come now!" said the Logothete. "Nobody questions an agent of the Post!"

Once more, Michael raised an eyebrow. "At least...not certain agents of the Post." His own position was not so exalted as Bourtzes'.

Both Varangians threw back their heads and laughed.

Psellus managed a thin smile. "That's the way of things."

The Logothete scowled. "Now, Michael, your circumstances are not so bad."

"Forgive me." Michael bowed his head, but he saw his superior's contorted face in his mind's eye. It was understandable that he disliked Michael's jest, but—

Still, Blachernites must have told the truth about the

contents of Bourtzes's saddlebags. Persons other than he had recovered the horse. But what if he'd seized the dispatch earlier...say, in the beech grove?

Chapter 9

The next morning, as soon as Michael arrived at the Great Palace, he headed for the ancient building called the Daphne and presented himself at the apartments of Nicetas Saponas, Rector of the Imperial household.

"He's out, probably stuffing his belly in the kitchens," the Varangian at the door informed him.

Michael suppressed a laugh. From what he'd heard about Saponas, that rang true. "Since he's out, I'd like to have a look at his rooms."

The guard shrugged. He wasn't about to stand in the way of the Post. "His office is just inside."

Michael stepped into a light, airy chamber with two casement windows overlooking an enclosed courtyard. A brightly patterned Persian carpet covered most of the marble floor, which radiated a warmth Michael could feel through his boots. Saponas was privileged enough to have a working hypocaust.

Along the walls lay several low cabinets, but a desk with carved-wood trim, adorned with a slipper-shaped oil lamp, dominated the chamber. Michael approached it and thumbed through several weighted stacks of parchments arranged there. There were purchase orders for both fresh foods and staples for the several Palace kitchens, inventories of supplies obtained for each suite of Imperial apartments, and lists of cooks, domestics, and other employees. Stephen's name was at the bottom of one of these.

In the desk's side compartments, Michael found only

pens, penknives, and ink pots. There was no sign of the missing dispatch.

Next Michael opened the cabinets, though clouds of dust immediately challenged him. After stifling a sneeze or two, he covered his mouth and nose with his handkerchief and leafed through the parchments stored there. They were all accounts from past years.

He moved the cabinets but found nothing. There were no telltale seams in the flooring. Grumbling in exasperation, he examined the undersides of the desk and chair and peered under the rug—in vain.

Now he turned to the door to Saponas's living quarters and entered, finding himself in a sitting room whose most prominent feature was a mosaic floor. Pale November sunlight streamed in through several arched windows, playing on the floor scene, depicted in colored glass and stone: a group of mounted noblemen and their hunting cheetahs charged after a gazelle.

The rest of the furnishings were also typical of a wealthy man's apartments: a curve-backed couch piled high with silk cushions, a few carved chairs, a dining table inlaid with ivory, and a low chest along the wall. Atop it were several goblets, a gold ewer, and a large clay bottle whose cork was still sealed with pitch.

Michael flipped up the lid of the ewer and sniffed its contents. Of course—a fragrant, sweetish wine. The head of His Majesty's household would hardly settle for swill.

The cabinet itself was empty except for a few extra pillows, which Michael pinched and poked, thoroughly, repeating the process with those on the couch. All of them contained only their feather stuffing.

Next Michael examined the bedchamber. As soon as he opened the door, the close, heavy smell of sweat and attar of roses assailed him. Once more he covered his nose and mouth with his handkerchief.

In the dim light, he could see drawers, fine wool hose, and a long silk tunic strewn about, on a thick Persian carpet. An unmade, rumpled bed lay against the far wall. On the wall above it was an icon of the Mother of God with an unlit vigil lamp hanging before it.

Michael was surprised that the maids hadn't tidied up yet, then reconsidered. They must know that Saponas was both slovenly and lenient and took advantage accordingly.

Michael crossed the room to a casement window, and flung open the drapes. In the sunlight, he poked at the mattress and shook out the bedclothes.

Nothing.

Dust motes swirled around him as he surveyed the room once more, finally resting his gaze on a large chest. When he lifted the lid, the pungent smell of cedar escaped. But the chest was filled with clothes, only with clothes.

He was about to leave when he realized he'd almost missed something: a narrow door of plain wood. Unlocked, it led into close, dust-filled gloom. He went to fetch the guard, and a lamp, and returned.

To all appearances, it was a storeroom without windows, with no ventilation. Some grimy, smelly underdrawers had been tossed on the floor, while several pairs of boots and sandals formed an irregular line upon one wall. In one corner stood a pair of unstrung hunting bows, as well as a bow-case and a quiver with twenty arrows. Each of these was marked with a broad black band.

What of it? Saponas, evidently a sometime recreational hunter, had a legitimate reason for possessing such equipment. In any case, all of it was covered with a residue of gritty dust.

Michael had had enough. "You say the Rector is in the kitchens?" he asked the guard. "Which ones?"

"He didn't bother to tell me. Probably at the Chrysotriclinium, where the Emperor is currently in residence."

Michael set out from the Daphne. He passed the gilded portals to the Chrysotriclinium—the Golden Throne Room—then paused in front of a side door guarded by two strapping Varangians.

One of the guards recognized him and waved him in. "You're here to see His Majesty?" he asked.

"No. I'm looking for the Rector."

"Go through the courtyard and look for the door behind the cypress trees."

"Thank you.' Michael cut through the anteroom to a garden containing a small pavilion and beds of bare, well-pruned rose bushes. On the far side a row of bare trees screened off a stucco-covered building. A hot, steamy smell, accompanied by the clank and clatter of dishes, came from behind it."

When Michael reached the building, he edged along the wall, stopping just outside an open door. The scent of wood smoke and onions and the sound of several voices drifted towards him.

He cast a furtive glance through the doorway, into a hazy, cavernous kitchen hung with an assortment of, pots, pans, and smoked meats. A graybeard was chopping onions at a rough-hewn table, while a woman clad in a colorless, stained garment, stirred a steaming pot over a fire. Wisps of white hair had escaped from beneath her kerchief.

They were not alone. A somewhat younger man, with longish, sandy hair, stood with his broad back towards Michael. "All I know is that His Majesty wants six young chickens for tomorrow," he said. "He and the Augusta are having a private party."

The elderly woman looked about to spit. No doubt she thoroughly disapproved of the Emperor's young mistress. At the same time, the graybeard looked up from his onions. "Where does he expect us to find anything young at this time of year?"

Their tormentor replied with an exaggerated shrug, which, on his portly frame, resembled an earthquake. "Find what you can and marinate it. Do what you have to do."

The old man scowled.

"Don't blame me," said the stout man. "I only work here—and take orders."

Michael nodded; this must be Saponas.

The old woman confirmed his guess. "Not...so!" she sputtered. "You come in here every day and demand bird's milk from us."

Saponas crossed to the hearth. "Come now, my dear, it can't be that bad," he said, patting her on the buttocks.

She froze. "For shame!"

The graybeard, presumably her husband, whirled

around and showed Saponas his fist.

Michael doubted that this was the first time that the Rector had taken such liberties.

"Come, come, I meant no harm," put in Saponas, now merely pinching her. "Go out to the markets—or send your assistants if your aches and pains won't permit. I'll give you money, and if you slip the vendor a little extra—hee, hee!"

The old man had seen the pinch. "Why you—" he muttered.

Michael wondered if Saponas were drunk, clowning, or playacting. He found the man's outrageous conduct fascinating.

Just at that moment, Saponas turned towards the doorway. He had a broad, fair face—Michael saw—and a beard that needed trimming. Still oblivious to Michael's presence, he eyed a hanging string of sausages and chopped one off with a kitchen knife. "Not bad," he said, between bites.

"Sir," began the old woman. "Today's Wednesday. You ought to fast."

Saponas guffawed. "I ought to. Of course, there's many things I ought to do. Why don't you hit me over the head with the Ten Commandments while you're at it? I daresay those tablets would carry—er—a bit more weight."

The graybeard waved his knife at Saponas. "How dare you?"

Michael, far from being shocked, was puzzled. He had the feeling that Saponas was trying to be as offensive as possible.

As though guessing Michael's thoughts, Saponas threw

back his head and laughed until he began to cough. It took him a short while to catch his breath. "It's high time I was on my way," he said, wiping his eyes. "Your damned onions are making me cry."

"Good riddance," said the old woman.

Saponas turned towards her—to make a rude gesture, Michael presumed. As he swung away from her, towards the door, she glared after him.

Only now did he notice Michael. He stopped short, his reddened eyes widening.

"Nicetas Saponas?" Michael showed the man his signet ring. "I'm Michael Taronites from the Post. I have some questions to ask you. Can we talk privately?"

Saponas's jaw dropped. "The Post? Shit! If you people want to talk to me, I must be in trouble." He laughed. "Tell me—what have I done?"

Michael glowered at him. "This is a serious matter."

"Oh."

Michael took advantage of the awkward moment to size up the former soapmaker. Again, he wondered if the man were drunk or simply clowning. He did smell of wine, and his florid face indicated that he drank more than was good for him. But though his hair and beard were in disarray, his gray eyes, steady despite their veined redness, belied his foolery.

He did appear healthy enough, aside from the ravages of drink on his face, and there were few strands of gray in his fair hair. He couldn't be much over forty.

"Let's go across the courtyard," said Saponas, now quite matter-of-fact. "There's a sitting room."

Michael followed him into a small, dusky chamber and chose to sit in a carved teakwood chair. Sighing deeply, the Rector sank onto a cushioned bench opposite him. Its joints creaked as he leaned back, patting his belly. "Now wait," he began. "I knew I'd heard your name before. You're the one that sent that little bugger to me yesterday."

"He needed work. And he knows nothing of the events I wish to discuss with you. At the time—neither did I. I didn't send him to spy on you."

"So, what do you want with me? Let's have it."

Michael found him irritating. "Sir, I repeat, this is an extremely serious matter."

Saponas dramatically slumped his shoulders. "Oh. What seems to be the trouble?"

"You're aware that Eustathios Bourtzes, an agent of the Post, was found murdered yesterday morning?"

Saponas widened his bloodshot eyes, then blinked. "Oh yes, I heard. A dreadful business!" he added, crossing himself hastily.

"Very."

Saponas lowered his head, resting his unkempt beard on his chest. What, if anything, was he thinking?

"Ah—"

"Yes? You were acquainted with him?"

Saponas looked up at the ceiling. "Just barely."

"Hm." Michael frowned. This was only partially true. Bourtzes had insulted him to his face. "But you were present at the highly secret meeting where Bourtzes's mission to the western province was discussed. You knew what he was doing there."

Saponas's mouth went slack.

"Did you have any reason to oppose his activities?"

"Why, no!"

"And how did you come to be at that meeting, anyway? You're hardly one of His Majesty's high counselors."

"His Majesty allowed me to be there. We had some...plans afterwards."

What "plans"? A drink fest or a gourmand's marathon? "Ah—was the time of Bourtzes's return discussed at that conference."

"No. He was to take as long as he needed."

Well! That squared with what Michael knew. But now he cleared his throat. "Now, listen: though you claim you hardly knew Bourtzes, we have evidence that the two of you didn't get along."

"That's nonsense."

"You're saying that he didn't call you a coarse buffoon, or something of the sort?"

Saponas flinched.

"But since, as you say, that's not the case, you won't mind telling us where you were night before last."

"I don't think you want to know where I was," he replied, winking.

"I see. What's the name of this...establishment?"

"Listen, I wasn't in a whorehouse. But I'm not a complete cad, to besmirch the reputation of a lady of good family."

"So, when did you arrive there?"

"Around sundown, Monday night."

"And when did you part company? Obviously in time to

be back here Tuesday morning, to interview applicants for employment."

"Um—yes."

"Still, I have only your word that you were with a lady."

Without replying, Saponas looked away. He pulled a none-too-clean silk handkerchief from his belt pouch and blew his nose loudly. Only then did he speak. "I'm sorry I can't be of more help."

"I'm sorry too."

Chapter 10

After leaving Saponas, Michael, set off for the Imperial Cabinet. The *Kanikleios* or Custodian of the Imperial Inkstand had an office here.

The *Kanikleios* was perhaps the most fortunate of courtiers. Though he had no staff of his own—as did the Logothete of the Dromos, the First Secretary, and others of high rank—and though his only official duty was to hold the pot of purple ink with which the Emperor signed his letters and decrees, he was permitted access to the Autocrator at any time of the day or night. Other dignitaries with the right to report directly to the Emperor were obliged to make an appointment.

But today the gilded double doors of the Emperor's office were shut—and unguarded. If His Majesty were absent. Syropoulos, the *Kanikleios,* might not be in the adjacent office.

Nevertheless, Michael knocked at his single width arched door and was pleased to find a response.

"Who goes there?"

Michael startled. The voice from within was euphonious, yet haughty.

"It's Taronites, from the Post. I have some questions for you."

"For *me?* Let's see what you have to say for yourself. Come in."

Michael winced. The man was incredibly arrogant. Still, he opened the door and found himself in a spacious chamber with a patterned carpet on the floor. Light from two arched windows rained down on the gilded bronze dog—the Inkstand—and on a massive sandalwood desk. Though it was midday, a lamp hanging over the bookstand burned perfumed oil.

Leo Syropoulos's black, well-combed head of hair was bent over a book. A fine gold chain, the sort that held a pectoral cross, glinted at his neckline. Gold. Of course—only the best for this fellow.

"Ahem—I beg your pardon," said Michael.

Syropoulos looked up. A scowl crossed his olive-skinned face as he smoothed his graying beard. "What do you want?"

The musky scent of the perfumed oil filled Michael's nostrils. "You know that one of our agents was found murdered yesterday?"

Syropoulos crossed himself with a sweeping gesture. "Bourtzes—I know. But what does that sordid affair have to do with me? What right does it give you to come barging in here?

Michael had thought of a good retort. "I came in because you told me to."

"An insolent fellow, aren't you?" Syropoulos picked up a small brass handbell from his desk. "Guard!"

"I think you'll find the guards on my side now," said Michael. "Instead of yelling, you'd best keep your strength—and your wits—for my questions."

"What questions?" Syropoulos rose and strode over to the windows, turning Michael his back. "I have nothing to do with this business."

"But you do. You were at the conference where

Bourtzes's mission to Philippopolis was planned. Besides His Majesty, the only others present were the Logothete of the Dromos and the Rector."

Syropoulos's broad shoulders remained as motionless as a mountain range. "That scum! He crashed the meeting!"

"Yes, the situation was regrettable."

A faint tremor crossed the other man's formidable back.

Good! Michael had his attention. "I'm sure you recall what was discussed."

Syropoulos did not speak at once. "We discussed the impending investigation of the Bogomils."

"Did anyone at that conference sympathize with them?"

Syropoulos spun around. "With that rabble? I should say not!"

Michael flinched involuntarily and stepped back. Syropoulos was slightly taller and definitely more muscular. "I'm not surprised."

Still, he did not hesitate to test the man. "Ah—do you recall the date set for Bourtzes's return?"

Syropoulos narrowed his eyes but came no closer. "Why you—That wasn't mentioned at all. We thought he'd be gone about six weeks, but he had permission to take as long as he needed."

Well, the man had seen through his ruse, but Michael could save the situation. "Well, good. Your account of the meeting matches those I've already heard. So, I'm sure you won't mind telling me where you were Monday night."

Blood rushed into Syropoulos's face. "You're implying that I killed Bourtzes? What nonsense!" His voice rattled the window glass.

"I'm sorry, but I'm obliged to ask these questions."

"If you really want to know, I was at home. My family and my servants will vouch for me."

"I'm sure they will. We'll interview them."

Once more Syropoulos turned away. This time he returned to his chair and his book. "Now, be good enough to go."

"I will," said Michael. "But I'll be back." He couldn't resist the impulse to peer over Syropoulos's shoulder; he was reading the *Iliad.*

Who, Michael wondered, was the man's favorite hero? Achilles, for his pride?

§

Once outside, Michael turned onto a walkway leading to the Post and pondered this morning's interviews. Arrogance seemed a part of Syropoulos's character, just as coarse buffoonery seemed a part of Saponas's. So far Michael could not tell if either man was hiding something.

Of course, the sooner he found out, the better. His step quickened as he approached the entrance to the Post.

"Michael, do slow down!" The familiar, pompous voice came from behind him.

Michael looked back and saw Psellus, who caught up to him in a few long strides.

"Any new developments?" asked Michael.

"Nothing much. But where have you been all morning?"

"Questioning that fool Saponas and Syropoulos too. This afternoon I must see the Court physician." *And Olympia.* Expectation, then impatience formed tight coils inside him.

Psellus jarred him back to the present. "So, you questioned those two. Did you learn anything?" He laughed—a tinny sound.

"Neither of them owns up to anything, which of course proves nothing. I did search Saponas's office and living quarters but found nothing suspicious."

Psellus turned serious. Gnawing on his mustaches, he fixed his dull brown eyes on Michael, then abruptly looked away. After a long pause, he spoke. "I have something rather...awkward to ask you."

"Awkward?"

"Yes." Psellus examined his booted feet. "There's one person you shouldn't forget to question. I mean—a person who was present at that meeting." Psellus, the eloquent orator, was suddenly tongue-tied.

Of course, Michael knew whom he meant. He'd understood Psellus's anxious behavior last night, and he had his own suspicions. "You mean the Logothete of the Dromos... Only, why?" He threw up his hands.

"I don't want to believe it, and I admit it's not likely," said Psellus. "Blachernites has always seemed an upright soul. But who knows what sort of double life he might lead? It wouldn't be the first time anyone—"

"I understand."

"And who else could have known the time of Bourtzes's return?" Psellus demanded.

"But I gather that no date was set."

"Still, there's a possibility that there was, but the date was known only to the Logothete."

"He would know, if anyone did. But I hope we're both

wrong."

Psellus set his lips. "Yes."

"I think we need to have his house searched and his household questioned—politely, of course," said Michael. "And his office should be inspected when he's not there. Likewise, Saponas's house in town should be examined, as well as Syropoulos's office and residence. I'll make arrangements with the Varangians."

"That's right. We must be thorough."

Michael felt a twinge of resentment. This is *my* investigation, Psellus!

After a moment's silence, he spoke again. "I still need to speak with Tripsychos. I know that he was in a very public fight with Bourtzes, but I don't quite understand the enmity between them."

"At one time, they both loved the same woman."

"And she married Bourtzes," said Michael.

"Yes."

"I'll plan to question him, then, and have his house searched."

"I'm sure His Majesty will be pleased with your progress," said Psellus, pensively scratching his beard.

"Oh—I almost forgot what I was supposed to tell you. Your—ah—friend, the Patriarch, left a message with us."

"He did?" Psellus, Michael knew, did not get along with the Patriarch.

"After the noon recess, he wants to see you—about what he terms a most urgent matter."

74

Chapter 11

When the mechanical clock in the Augusteum rang out the seventh hour of the day, Michael crossed the square and headed for the back door of the Patriarchate. For the present, he would put aside his wish to see Olympia. If the Patriarch had summoned Michael, Michael would go. At one time, the Patriarch had protected Michael from arrest.

Once inside, Michael stepped into a dimly-lit corridor. A servant emerged from the shadows and escorted him upstairs, then knocked on an arched oaken door. "Your Holiness, His Honor Lord Taronites is here."

For a moment, Michael thought that the servant referred to some other person, then understood that he was the one referred to.

"Admit him, please," came a resonant voice from within the chamber.

Inside, Michael paused on the worn carpet. A dark-bearded man, tall and well-proportioned, rose from his desk. Though simply clad in monk's habit and cap, he was Michael Cerularius, chief bishop of the Church of Constantinople. Only the icon on a heavy gold chain around his neck indicated his episcopal rank.

"Last night I heard that you had returned," he said.

Michael accepted his blessing and kissed his hand.

"And so, you sent for me?" He noticed a bulging vein on the Patriarch's brow.

"Please sit down." The Patriarch sank into his chair and, letting out a long sigh, pensively fingered his chain.

Michael pulled up a chair on the other side of the desk, facing the arched windows that overlooked the Palace rooftops: domes, vaults, and gables covered with gold or lead. "Your Holiness, what can I do for you?"

The Patriarch's dark eyes met his. "You said once that you hoped that there was some way you could be of aid to me..."

Michael all but jumped up. "Oh, yes, Your Holiness, I'd be only too glad."

"I realized that they've put you on the case of this unfortunate Bourtzes..." He paused, crossing himself. "God rest his soul. I'm supposed to preside at his funeral tomorrow—down the street, so to speak, at Hagia Eirene... But I digress. I do need your help, though not for myself. I know that Father Zosimas of the Studion is very dear to you."

"He is. As a matter of fact, I saw him yesterday."

The Patriarch's eyes half-closed. "Ah, then you *know*."

Michael's eyes widened. "Know what? I know nothing. He didn't—" Sitting on the edge of his chair, he studied the Patriarch's swarthy face, now set in lines of anguish.

Vague suspicions swept over Michael. "Just what's going on?" he asked. And now these suspicions became images flashing through his mind: Blachernites acting surprised, almost shocked, when Michael said he planned to visit Zosimas; unknown persons flitting through the halls at the Studion; and, finally, Zosimas's reticence about his recent activities. And his strange remark: "Perhaps I should have been a soldier."

"What's wrong?"

The Patriarch's broad shoulders slumped. "I see. You really haven't heard. Well, you only just returned."

"I came home Monday night, only to find a domestic crisis awaiting me. Then I collapsed from exhaustion. And yesterday morning the Varangians dragged me straight off to the murder scene. So Bourtzes's case has completely occupied me."

"So, of course you haven't heard," said the Patriarch, straightening himself. Deep creases marred his brow. "Well, I'll tell you now. Several persons have brought charges of immorality against our dear Father Zosimas: specifically, charges of indecent behavior and lying with men."

Michael sprung to his feet. "That's nonsense!"

The Patriarch raised his eyes; Michael noticed that they were weary and reddened. "Yes, of course it's nonsense, but the problem is that the plaintiffs appear to be credible. So, we've opened an investigation which could proceed to a full ecclesiastical trial."

Michael dropped into his chair. "Mother of God, save us!"

"I'm sure you can understand that this course of action is the wisest. If we simply dismiss the charges, people will accuse us of shielding him—or even of participating in his alleged crimes. And—strictly as a formality, you understand—I've suspended him from the priesthood until he's been vindicated. I have no doubt that he will be."

"I'll prove those people are lying," said Michael, digging his fingernails into his palms. "I'll find some way to destroy their testimony."

The Patriarch's frown relaxed, and the dark vein on his

brow almost disappeared. "Why, Michael, I didn't dare hope... That's exactly what I was going to ask you."

Michael kept his hands clenched, to keep them from shaking. "I could do no less for him. I wasn't able to help my father when he needed it, but this time I'll—"

The Patriarch nodded. "Yes, you've known him all your life. So, you will bear witness to his good character in court?"

"Of course! And as I said, I'll do more than that."

"Well, at least we have many people willing to testify on his behalf. Thank God for that."

"Alas, I understand now." Michael spoke in a hollow tone.

"Understand what?"

"Yesterday, when I went to see Father in the scriptorium, he seemed both agitated and fatigued. Also, someone was lurking in the corridor."

"Spying on him, no doubt, trying to find out if he was doing anything else...inappropriate, or trying to keep him from it."

"But who's behind this, and why?"

A baleful light shone in the Patriarch's eyes. "Who? You'll see. As to why—we don't know. God willing, you can find out."

"I'll do my best."

The Patriarch leaned back in his chair. "Unfortunately, this sort of scandal-mongering is rather common among churchmen."

"Really?"

"Oh, yes. And the victim of such slanders is usually

someone like Zosimas: a person of many gifts and talents, a person with strong opinions—in short—a person one either loves or hates. And those who hate him are often envious of his aforementioned gifts and the favor he enjoys. Don't forget: Zosimas belongs to a prominent family, and if he weren't a monk, he'd be a high Court official or a professor. Certain people resent such things."

"I'm sure."

"Sometimes, though, there's more than mere envy at stake. Sometimes they disagree with the poor man's theology. But whatever the case, they try to concoct some accusation."

"I think I understand."

"Of course, some charges are easy to prove false," said the Patriarch. "You can't accuse someone of stealing money from the Church if the funds are right there in the treasury. But morals charges are much harder to disprove. So, if a clergyman is married, his enemies say he's committed adultery. If he's a monk, they say he…likes men."

Michael grimaced. "And you say this sort of thing is common?"

The Patriarch's expression softened. "I'm sorry. I've scandalized you."

"I suppose I shouldn't be shocked. Monks and clergy are only human."

"But one expects more from those who have dedicated their lives to God."

"Yes." Michael bowed his head. "One can't help but be upset."

He looked up again. "So just who is accusing Zosimas?"

"Take a look." The Patriarch gestured towards some parchments on the desk. "These are the written statements submitted by his accusers. He's been given copies of them and is now preparing his defense."

"He is?" Had Zosimas been working on that just before Michael had come by and seen him cleaning out his desk?

The Patriarch rose slowly, as though it pained him. "Please! Sit in my chair." He indicated the documents again, then withdrew to the window, and looked out on the square. But Michael did not doubt that his mind was working steadily.

Though embarrassed, he moved to the Patriarch's chair and pulled the first accusation towards him.

The plaintiff was a certain Peter of Serrhes, a grocer with a shop and residence in the Street of the Peacock. He was writing on behalf of his cousin and house guest Luke, a visitor from the provinces. According to Peter's testimony, Luke, an eighteen-year-old shepherd from Macedonia, had, in the company of other shepherds, journeyed to Mount Athos a year and some months ago for the purpose of trade.

Peter proceeded to remind his readers that such contacts are one of the few necessary ties that the monks of Athos maintain with the outside world. Since they do not engage in animal husbandry and keep no female beasts, they must import such cheese and wool as they need.

Thus, young Luke and his companions made the rounds of the Athonite monasteries. Once or twice, though, the youth allegedly became separated from the others and lost his way in the thick forests that cover most of the mountain. On one of these occasions, he stumbled upon a hermitage, where the monks offered him both their humble hospitality and a chance for him to sell his wares.

The settlement, known as the skete of the Prophet Moses, consisted of perhaps five or six monks, each living in a hut or cave within reasonable vicinity of a chapel. At the time that Luke was there, the monks had a visitor from "outside:" Father Zosimas, a monk of the Studion in Constantinople. He had received a blessing from his abbot to retire to the Holy Mountain for a time in order to pray.

According to Peter of Serrhes, the unfortunate Luke was lodged in the same "guest house" or house as Zosimas, "who had nothing monastic about him but his habit. This false monk," wrote Peter, "seduced my young cousin Luke and made him do the most lude things," all of which he described in the frankest terms.

Michael crumpled the accusation in his fist. He couldn't stand to read it to the end. He raised his hand to throw it into the brazier that heated the room, then stopped himself. He would not destroy evidence, even though the least offensive thing in the letter was Peter's atrocious spelling.

"Peter of Serrhes is not an educated man," said the Patriarch. "He doesn't know how to put things delicately. As a matter of fact, I'm surprised he can write."

"And he wrote lies," said Michael, slamming the parchment on the desk. As an afterthought, he tried to press out the wrinkles with his fingertips. "But he could have found someone to write this filth for him."

"No doubt."

"I wonder, though..." Michael began. "It's true that Father Zosimas retired to a hermitage on Mt. Athos a year ago last summer. How did these evil tongues find out?"

The Patriarch turned back from the window, his eyes wide and sorrowful. "Come now! Anyone who wanted to know could have learned that."

"Do these people have a connection with the Studion?"

The Patriarch nodded. "They might. You'll see."

"I wish we could go to the Holy Mountain and interview people, to see if they remember Luke." Michael sighed long and deeply, for such a journey was clearly impossible. In fair weather, it took a good ten days overland, but now the mountain passes were clogged with snow. And also, the seas were rough.

"And we should settle this affair by the middle of next week," said the Patriarch, twisting his mouth. "Under the circumstances, it's not proper to suspend Zosimas for a longer time. But even if we could talk to people on Athos, there's a good chance that they might not remember Luke, assuming he did go there."

"True. In fact, do we have any proof that he and Peter are related?"

"Only Peter's word."

"Which I'll try to prove isn't worth much."

The Patriarch's dark eyes narrowed. "Unfortunately, Peter appears to be a reputable man. And don't forget— we've received other accusations as well."

Michael exhaled in exasperation. "Written by whom?" He was beginning to feel helpless—just as when he had been accused of murder.

The Patriarch came over and stood at Michael's back. "One is from Matthew, a novice at the Studion. He's also quite young—about eighteen—and according to the Abbot, of good character. But of course, the Abbot himself will testify for Zosimas." He slid Matthew's statement towards Michael, who read it clenching the sides of the page.

"So! Matthew accuses Zosimas of making indecent advances to him while they were working alone in the scriptorium...advances which, of course, he repulsed."

"An act that would absolve him of all guilt—if his allegations were true."

Michael faced the Patriarch. "Who—and what—was Matthew before he entered the monastery?"

"The Abbot says that he's from the country, but he'd been living in the City with his aunt and uncle. They're tradespeople."

Michael cocked an eyebrow. "Grocers?"

"No. I think the Abbot said they're weavers."

"Why was he staying with them? Is he an orphan?"

"That I don't know. Ask him at the trial."

"I'll ask him that—and much more!"

The Patriarch indicated a third parchment on the desk. "Here's the last one."

It was written by a certain Priestmonk Jonas, a member of the Monastery of the Studion for over fifteen years. He claimed that one night after Compline, he was taking a walk around the grounds and heard untoward noises in one of the writing rooms. He found the door to the building unlocked, so he went in and stole down the hall towards the commotion...towards the scriptorium where Zosimas worked. Then, without warning, Jonas flung open the door. Though the room was dark, he distinguished Zosimas's form—and that of another monk. Jonas could not identify the latter for the simple reason that both Zosimas and his lover bolted out the open casement window.

"Lover! Who is this liar?" For a moment Michael regarded the brazier.

"Unfortunately for Zosimas, he's a credible witness." The Patriarch's face twisted, as though in pain. "As he says, he's been a monk at the Studion for a long time. The Abbot describes him as a man of high moral character and a very strict manner of life."

"I wonder," said Michael. He got up and paced the floor. Something was tugging at the back of his mind. "What's his background, and where is he from?"

"He's from a noble family that's resided here in the City for generations. I believe that his father was a member of the Senate, though, to tell the truth, I have no idea whether or not his parents are still living."

"They must own estates in the provinces," said Michael, considering a certain possibility.

The Patriarch frowned as he tried to recall what he knew about the family. "I believe his surname is Attaleiates. So, they're from the city of Attaleia in Anatolia, at least originally."

"Oh." This was not the connection Michael had been hoping for.

The Patriarch regained his own chair, pushing aside the three accusations as if they were so much rubbish. Michael sat down across from him.

"There is something curious about Jonas's statement," said the Patriarch.

"Oh?"

"Peter of Serrhes had his accusation delivered directly to our offices two Saturdays ago, while the Novice Matthew gave his to the Abbot who in turn forwarded it to me. This was about a week ago. However, Jonas gave his to the Abbot two days later."

"Yes, that's curious. But there's also something odd about Jonas's story. Why should the window have been open at a time when the scriptorium was not in use? And would people doing something illicit have opened it??"

"No."

"Also, Your Holiness, when did this alleged crime take place? Matthew claims that Zosimas approached him at the beginning of October, but Jonas specifies no time."

The Patriarch nodded. "So, we'll ask him."

"Will he say that this incident only just took place, or will he say it happened some time ago?"

"In the latter case, he'll insist he said nothing, trying to cover Zosimas's sins, but since the scandal was now out in the open, he decided he might as well speak up."

"I gather it *is* out in the open." Michael recalled Blachernites's odd look, when he'd mentioned Zosimas.

"You've been away, so you don't know. But yes, it is being discussed in every square, market stall, bath-house, and wine shop. Of course, I've denounced all slanderers from the pulpit, and I've advised our priests that they should lay severe penances on anyone spreading vicious gossip about a man who hasn't even been tried. But nobody's going to speak of these things in front of a priest."

Michael thought for a moment. "Do you think that

certain people are intentionally spreading these rumors, or are they simply passing from mouth to mouth?"

The Patriarch threw up his hands. "I don't know!"

Michael closed his eyes and felt hot tears behind them. Had he cared for himself so much, when he had been accused? No doubt. Whom did one love more than one's self? But he did love Zosimas and believed in his innocence. "You do believe...?"

"Of course, I think he's innocent! What I don't understand is why they're out to discredit him." He rested his bearded chin in his hands. "Or, perhaps I do have an idea, but it's rather far-fetched."

"Really?"

"Over the past several months I've received letters from certain prominent citizens in Macedonia—more precisely from the environs of Philippopolis—and also from several bishops in that area. All these people request that Father Zosimas be consecrated Archbishop of Philippopolis, the old archbishop having reposed in the Lord last summer."

Michael startled at the mention of that city and jumped to his feet. "Of course! That's just the connection I was looking for. I wondered if Father Jonas's family was from Macedonia. It seems that Matthew's family is, and Peter of Serrhes most certainly is."

"Most people back there remember Zosimas fondly, even though he's spent most of his life in Constantinople. Aside from his own virtues, it's on account of his family."

"Exactly," Michael put in. "The Vladislavichi, or at least the branch of the family in those parts, are well-liked by high officials and peasants alike. Nobody seems to mind

86

that they're of Slavonic descent, or that one of their ancestors was the chief of his tribe."

The Patriarch looked up. "It would appear that our grocer has no use for them."

"And I'm sure there are others who do not wish to see Zosimas as the local bishop."

"I was thinking of the Bogomils," said the Patriarch.

"So was I." Their eyes met. "In fact, I'll tell you something that's privileged information, or at least it was."

The Patriarch leaned toward him, a dark fire in his eyes. "Yes?"

"Bourtzes was sent to Philippopolis to investigate the Bogomils, to uncover their seditious activities, if any. And a certain person at Court believes that the Bogomils may have killed him."

The Patriarch drew a quick breath.

"Are there Bogomils here in the City?"

"I'm sure. But they know how to hide."

"Now, this is what I fear: the local Bogomils are trying to discredit Father Zosimas, to prevent him from becoming Archbishop of Philippopolis."

"That is possible, at the very least. And now that I hear that from you..."

Michael returned to his chair and inclined his head in thought. "You've encouraged me. And now I wonder: do Father Zosimas's accusers have something to do with Bourtzes's death?"

The Patriarch threw up his hands again. "I don't see how they could have actually murdered him, but they may be involved. As it is, we'll have trouble enough proving that

Peter of Serrhes and the others are Bogomils."

"True." Michael slumped his shoulders. Indeed, this theory was preposterous. Who, of his list of suspects for Bourtzes's murder, could possibly be a Bogomil? Metiga, a heathen Patzinak who followed the gods of his people? The haughty Leo Syropoulos? He appeared to consider the Bogomil heresy the most odious bad manners, if nothing worse. And Blachernites, Logothete of the Dromos? The man was known for his scorn for all old-wives' tales and heresies.

What other possibilities existed? Gregory Tripsychos, Bourtzes's rival in love? Michael knew nothing of his beliefs—not yet. And finally, there was Nicetas Saponas, to all appearances a buffoon, a glutton, and a drunkard. Could a man with unbridled appetites and a taste for obscene jokes belong to a sect that condemned the physical world as the work of the devil? From what Michael had heard of the Bogomils' moral habits, only a few led a strict life. The rest were guilty of everything from excessive eating and drinking to utter licentiousness.

Again, Michael's eyes met the Patriarch's. "Is there a connection. I don't know yet. But I'll do my best for Father Zosimas."

The Patriarch arose and placed a fatherly hand on Michael's shoulder. "Please do. It's extremely difficult to overturn the decisions of an ecclesiastical court. But even if the charges can't be proved…"

"He'll be under a cloud."

"Exactly. We must expose his accusers as liars and dishonorable men."

"In which case I shouldn't be sitting here. I'll investigate the plaintiffs as soon as possible, but this afternoon I must see the Court physician."

"And the lady?" The Patriarch raised a heavy eyebrow.

Michael felt the blood rush to his face. "Excuse me, Your Holiness, but what do you know about—?"

"I hear things." He smiled, and the act brightened his lined, austere countenance. "Besides, we're distant cousins. Didn't you know?"

Michael swallowed his embarrassment. "Um—I think I'd heard something to that effect."

The Patriarch walked him to the door. "Well, God go with you. We'll be in touch. The trial is set for Monday."

Michael kissed his hand and departed. He felt beads of sweat form on his brow. For though the Palace was clamoring for Bourtzes's murderer, he could not abandon Father Zosimas.

Chapter 12

The *bong* of the mechanical clock in the Augusteum could be heard in the Mangana Palace. "It's the ninth hour," said the Court physician, looking up from the parchments spread over his desk. "All you have to do now, Lady Olympia, is crush some hyssop and prepare a poppy-juice decoction. Then you can go home if you like."

Lady Olympia, who was sitting at the table by the windows, raise her blond head—gladly—from a volume of Galen. Despite the man's valuable insights into the structure and workings of the body, he was a pompous windbag. "Thank you, but I'm in no hurry. My servants won't be here for another hour at least." Still, she was not sorry to abandon Galen.

"I'll start on the medicine now." With a swish of her gray wool robe, she stood, pausing to pull up her matching kerchief, which had fallen back around her plaited, bound-up hair.

"Ah—all right." Acropolites was re-reading what he had just written, his final report on Bourtzes's death.

"Is something wrong, Your Excellency?"

"No." He rubbed his temples. "I'm just weary—that's all."

Olympia noticed the dark half-moons under his eyes and concluded that he was telling the truth—if only partially.

"Is it the Bourtzes case?"

"Oh—well—yes. I've made a list of the effects found on his body and in his saddlebags. There's a copy for

Taronites."

She felt herself flush but managed to keep her voice even. She had recovered from her terror that he might have been murdered. Now she only wished to see him.

"So am I, but he must be very busy."

"Oh, if only he's turned up something—"

"Yes. It was such a vicious thing...ah...well, never mind."

"What—that he was beaten, perhaps, and strangled. Certainly, it was a monster in human form that did it."

He looked away.

"Wait—you haven't told me everything, have you?"

Acropolites bowed his head. "Lady, you're better off not knowing."

"Was he...raped?"

Startled, the doctor sat up straight. "How did you—?"

Olympia averted her glance, for his sake as much as hers. "It was easy. What else could be so dreadful that you wouldn't want to tell me?"

Now the doctor blushed. "Lady, such filth isn't fit for your ears."

"But I'm a physician. Or at least, God willing, I soon will be."

§

Once the guards had admitted Michael to the Mangana, he quickened his pace and mounted the stairs two at a time. Only when he reached Acropolites's half-open door did he pause to catch his breath.

It occurred to him that this time he didn't need to fabricate an excuse to meet Olympia. This time he had a grisly murder to discuss with the doctor.

Not that he had anything to be ashamed of. Whenever Michael saw her, Acropolites was always standing nearby, sometimes participating in their conversations, sometimes smiling indulgently. The two or three of them spoke of Palace affairs, medicine, theology, even the poetry of the ancients. And of course, Michael and Olympia touched not at all, or only with their eyes. Who could find fault with such innocence?

Many people: chiefly the parents of young, unmarried women of good family. Their daughters' wishes were of no account.

We'll see about that! Michael thought. But what, he wondered, were the lady's wishes?

He put the thought aside and combed his hair into place with his fingers. "Good evening," he called.

Acropolites moved away from his desk, scraping his chair against the floor, and stood up. "Michael! It's good to see you."

He stepped into the room and heard the sudden clatter of pottery. Yet aside from the doctor, the office was empty. A single clay lamp burned on the desk; white darkness gathered in the corners.

"Lady Olympia is in the apothecary room. She'll be out soon."

The doctor spoke truly. Moments later, the door opened, and a heavy scent, sweetish but medicinal, drifted into the office. Olympia entered in its wake, carrying a taper. Her gold earrings, not covered by her kerchief, glinted in the lamplight. The downy hairs above her upper lip glistened.

Michael sucked in his breath. "Good evening," he managed to say, then bowed—a model of decorum.

She returned his greeting. Her eyes, the color of sandalwood, studied him. "Have you been well?" As she lit the rack of lamps near the table, she inclined her head, awaiting his reply.

"If could be better," he said, "if I knew who killed Bourtzes." *And if I could clear Father Zosimas. If I dared hope we could be together.*

Acropolites creased his smooth brow. "This is a thankless job, isn't it?"

Olympia's eyes widened in concern.

"However," said the doctor, "all we can do is apply ourselves to the task at hand."

The three of them moved towards the table. Michael sat down across from Acropolites, while Olympia settled herself at the far end, her back to the windows.

Acropolites pushed a sheet of parchment towards Michael. "This is your copy of the list of Bourtzes's effects."

Michael looked it over. "Wool cap and cloak," it read. "Wool tunic, linen undertunic and drawers, wool hose: all torn and/or soiled. Leather boots, somewhat worn. Dagger in sheath, belt pouch containing a few coppers, signet ring."

"His signet ring will be buried with him," said the doctor.

"I hear his funeral is tomorrow. Are you going?" asked Michael.

"Probably."

"I will too."

"Afterwards, I'll call on his widow," put in Olympia. "I'll

return his belongings."

"Ah—good!" Michael spoke absent-mindedly; something about this list disturbed him. "What was in his saddlebags?" he asked. "Do you have a list of those items?"

The doctor pushed another parchment toward him. "Two complete changes of clothes, similar to the above. One long dress tunic—maroon wool. Comb, cake of soap. Official mail seized by the Post. Also, a bow, in a half-case, and a quiver containing thirty-five arrows." A double quiver contained forty.

"I see," said Michael although he didn't quite see what had happened to Bourtzes. "He's short five arrows—why? It appears that he was assaulted at close range and by surprise. He didn't even draw his dagger. No doubt he couldn't."

"He could have used five arrows to drive off wild beasts or brigands," said the doctor.

"True enough," said Michael. "But still, something isn't right here. He should have been carrying dispatches—those are missing. And he should have had more money. Was he killed for that? It doesn't seem right. Or, was he killed for his dispatches?"

"In any case," said the doctor, "our office is keeping these lists. We've given copies to you and to the Varangian Guard, and we'll give another set to Bourtzes's widow."

Michael scratched the nape of his neck. "Something is missing. Something still isn't right."

"We do have his signet ring," said Olympia. "If the murderer's intent was robbery, why didn't he take that?"

"I don't believe it was robbery," said Michael. "Something sinister, something wicked is going on here."

He slumped in his chair, suppressing a groan.

The physician took a long look at him and creased his brow again. "Michael, are you ill?"

"Some things make me ill," said Michael, staring at the smooth oak tabletop.

"Bourtzes's death?" asked the doctor.

Michael straightened himself in his chair. "Yes, but there's more. I—I've just come from the Patriarch's. He had to be the one to tell me about Father Zosimas."

"Oh, oh, oh!" said Acropolites.

"I saw Zosimas yesterday, and he told me nothing. I didn't know what was going on because I've been away, but it seems everybody else does."

Now Olympia spoke. "Not I. I don't know."

"Well, of course people would try to protect your ears from such filth," said the doctor.

She gave him an exasperated look.

Michael spoke up. "Evidently people are spreading gossip all over the City. The facts of the case are that certain people have leveled serious morals charges against Father Zosimas. His trial is set for Monday."

Her eyebrows came together. "But surely the charges are false. From what I've heard—"

"Of course, they're false! But now the Patriarch wants me to prove that they are."

"And will you?" asked the physician.

"Of course! I can't turn my back on him. He's...he's been like a father to me."

"What are they saying?" Olympia inquired.

Acropolites raised a restraining hand. "Lady, that talk

isn't fit for your ears."

"Again!" she glared at her teacher. "Honestly! As if I couldn't imagine…"

"Yes, really," said Michael. He felt his neck grow hot, but he admired Olympia's spirit.

"So," he concluded, "I'm taking on the monk's case, as well as Bourtzes's."

The doctor nodded. "Really? What have you—"

A sharp rap on the door started them all. The voice that followed it was accented but authoritative. "Taronites, are you here?"

Michael turned; Ingvar's hulking form, clad in the red tunic of the Varangian Guard, filled the doorway. "As you see," Michael said.

Ingvar strode across the room. Awkwardly bending his long legs, he sat down opposite Olympia. His face was ruddy from the cold, and his silver-blond hair shone in the lamplight.

"You wanted to see me?" asked Michael.

"Yes. I wanted to let you know that our men have searched the offices of George Blachernites, Leo Syropoulos, and Gregory Tripsychos—and found nothing suspicious. We also searched their houses. Again—nothing."

"Does Blachernites know you searched his premises?"

"He does, but our men made excuses—that Psellus was looking for a report that seemed to have gone missing."

"I see. Now, did you question these three directly?"

"Blachernites—yes. He was rather put out. And Syropoulos was insulted. We didn't find Tripsychos in his office or at home."

"I hear he was wounded," said Michael, "that he's ill now."

"Well, we didn't find him at home."

Michael raised an eyebrow. "So, what do Blachernites and Syropoulos have to say for themselves? Where were they Monday night?"

"We couldn't ask the Logothete directly, but he mentioned that he was home. But his wife is away, visiting a daughter who just gave birth."

"How convenient! Now what about Syropoulos?"

"His wife and servants claim he was home Monday night."

"Oh."

"And as for Tripsychos, his servants say he did leave the house on Monday night. He went to St. John's Hospital to have the dressing on his wound changed."

Michael bowed his head in thought. That made sense. But why didn't Tripsychos have himself admitted to the hospital, to recuperate in peace?

"So, we'll question the hospital personnel," he concluded. "Now—one last question. Did you search Saponas's house?"

"Yes, but Saponas's son said that Papa doesn't really live there anymore."

"His son..." Michael mused.

"He lives in the Street of the Soapmakers with his wife and servants," said Ingvar. "Like his father, he's a soapmaker. Unlike his father, he's a pleasant person, if you don't notice the scars all over his face."

The Court physician shrank. "Did he have smallpox?"

"Maybe." Ingvar shrugged off the dread disease and completed his report. "The younger Saponas says he can't vouch for his father's movements Monday night. Of course, that's not to say that the fool killed Bourtzes—just that he was nowhere near the family home."

Olympia gasped. "So all these people are under suspicion?"

"All these and more," said Michael.

"Now what about the savage?" asked Ingvar. "Have you visited his taverns yet?"

At first Michael did not grasp the Varangian's meaning. "You mean Metiga the Patzinak? No. I'll do that tonight."

"The Akolouthos thinks you should," said Ingvar. "He doesn't think the Patzinak was innocent of that business last winter. Who vouched for him? Madams, pimps, and whores—what sort of witnesses are they?"

Michael cast a withering glance at the Varangian. "Mind the lady!" If the Norseman considered Olympia a woman of easy virtue because she studied medicine and took some part in public life, Michael would show him. Then too, there were other things Michael didn't like about Ingvar's little speech. Who was in charge of this investigation? Michael or the Akolouthos?

Ingvar bowed his head. "I'm sorry, Your Ladyship."

Satisfied, Michael stole a glance at Olympia. In the yellow glow of the lamps, it was hard to tell. At last, she nodded. "I don't care for coarse language, but I've heard all the words."

"Lady Olympia has older brothers," said the physician.

"And older sisters," said Olympia. "They're even

worse."

"Is that so?" asked Michael, who had no siblings. He was glad of the momentary distraction from the case and his lack of progress.

Nevertheless, he returned to the business at hand. "I'll question the Patzinak tonight," he said. "And there's another possibility I need to explore: three men have brought accusations against Father Zosimas of the Studion—"

"Oh yes!" said Ingvar. "I heard about that monk. Do you think he—"

"No, he didn't," said Michael. "But it's strange that these things came to light around the time of Bourtzes's murder. The two cases could well be connected." He would need to provide a reason for his defense of Zosimas even as he worked on Bourtzes's case. Indeed, this theory might even prove to be true.

Chapter 13

By the time Michael left the Mangana Palace and started up the hill, the sky had turned a deep gray. The wooden gongs of the nearby churches had long since ceased ringing for Vespers.

A cold wind blew down from the north, whipping his hair into his face, shaking the bare-limbed trees that flanked the Mangana gates. He wiped his smarting eyes then donned the wool cap he'd stuck under his belt. Now he could go on; he must.

Only, how was he supposed to find Bourtzes's killer soon enough to please the authorities *and* clear Zosimas by Monday?

He knew what he must accomplish this evening: he would investigate the Patzinaks' favorite taverns. Hopefully he would find them as well.

But now the shadowy bulk of the Church of Hagia Eirene loomed on the ridge ahead of him. Light shone through the slit-like windows at the base of its dome. He remembered now: tomorrow was the feast day of St. John Chrysostom, Archbishop of Constantinople. The humble, the poor, and the virtuous had loved him, while the haughty and the wicked hated him.

Michael thought of Zosimas and wondered if things ever changed. Without making a conscious decision, he headed towards the church.

Both the outer and inner doors stood open, revealing rank upon rank of cramped humanity. Michael pulled off his cap and nudged his way through the narthex, into the back of the nave. As the warmth of the many bodies seeped into him, he loosened his cloak and breathed in the heavy, incense-laden air.

The service was almost over. "Vouchsafe, O Lord, to keep us this evening without sin," the reader intoned.

Sin? Did a few wine shops present any great temptation? He knew that the world provided far worse.

§

After stopping home to stuff down a hunk of bread and to pick up some money, Michael set out for the west side of the City, for Metiga the Patzinak's haunts. He tried the first few pothouses—on the north side of the Mese—without success, finding only obsequious proprietors and customers in various stages of intoxication. "No, Your Honor, I don't remember them," with an outstretched palm, or "Huh? They ain't been in here lately."

He had only one tavern left to check. To reach it, he crossed the Mese, leaving its widely-spaced lanterns behind, and headed down a murky byway.

Somewhere in a dark gap between buildings, a boot crunched gravel. Michael froze and forced himself to grasp the leather-wrapped hilt of his dagger.

He stared into the gloom. "Show yourself, coward!"

He was not surprised when no one appeared.

Finally, he sighted a hanging lantern and, bathed in its yellow glow, a carved wooden door. Fixed to the wall was a gilded bronze plaque with a gryphon in relief. So, this was one of the Patzinaks' haunts, the wine shop known as the Golden Gryphon.

Trying to get his bearings, Michael sidestepped a foul-smelling puddle and looked around. Though two-story houses lined this street and those adjoining it, the Gryphon faced open country.

§

Michael looked out past the jagged ruin of the old city wall. Rolling fields and farmlands spread out into a darkness pricked by a few points of light. Somewhere out there was the grove where they had found Bourtzes's corpse.

Shivering, Michael turned back to the tavern and went in.

It was exactly what he expected: high-class and high-priced. The stone floor looked freshly swept, and the chairs and tables were of solid, well-polished wood. Candles and hanging lamps lit the room—though not too brightly. A pair of large braziers provided sufficient warmth, though the charcoal fumes they exuded stung his nostrils.

The customers, dressed in garments of fine wool, talked quietly among themselves or played chess. Only a few high-pitched guffaws or giggles rose above the well-modulated conversation.

Two figures stood out. They wore fur caps atop their long black hair and untrimmed beards, and their brocades silk coats. Michael knew at once where he'd seen the green one.

He edged over to the counter. "Please, sir," he addressed, the stocky middle-aged proprietor, "bring me a cup of white wine, half full. And when I settle with my friends, bring us a pitcher of water and a jar of your best." The water was mostly for him—of course. He needed to keep his wits about him.

The tavern-keeper flinched, then put down the pewter cup he was wiping. "Ah—you must be new here. Or are you from—Listen, I usually close at seven…"

Michael smiled faintly; he rather doubted it. "Actually, I'm not from the police." He flashed his signet ring.

The proprietor shrank. "Whatever you say."

"We can talk later," said Michael. He slid some money across the counter, then picked up his cup—also pewter—and made his way to the Patzinaks' table. "Good evening, gentlemen. You must be the honorable Metiga and his most esteemed brother."

The Patzinaks stirred, exuding a stench of sweat and horses. Their love of civilized pleasures did not extend to frequent bathing.

Michael choked down a wave of nausea and reminded himself to breathe shallowly.

The nomad in the green coat bared white teeth in a broad smile. "Yes, I am Metiga," he said, with a heavy accent. "Who are you?"

"I'm Michael Taronites, from the Post."

Another smile, a brief pause. "Ah, what brings us the honor?"

"We need to talk. I'm having some wine sent over."

"As you wish. Here," he said, indicating his companion with a sweep of his yellowish, long-fingered hand. "This is my brother Uzun, really my half-brother. My father had many wives."

"I see." Michael nodded to Uzun, then slid into a chair opposite him. He kept his cup close to hand and sipped his wine slowly, while studying the Patzinaks.

Though Uzun was the younger and thinner of the two, they looked much alike. They had the same long black hair and beard, sallow skin, and good teeth. Metiga, however, was the handsomer. Uzun's broad-bridged nose spoiled his appearance.

Michael understood that both Patzinaks were far from stupid. Uzun seemed especially wary, observing Michael through his narrowed black eyes. He appeared about to speak when a waiter set a pottery wine jug and a pitcher in front of Michael.

He pushed the jug towards the Patzinaks. "Please, be my guests."

"We thank you," said Metiga, moving aside the crock they'd just emptied. "Here, I pour," he added, sloshing the red wine of Cyprus into his cup. He promptly served his brother, then extended the jug to Michael.

"No thank you. I prefer white." He pulled the pitcher close and hoped that they did not notice its true contents. He was glad the light was dim.

Metiga tossed of his wine, then leaned back and observed Michael for a moment. "What can we do for you?"

Michael set down his cup and leaned across the table. "I'm investigating the death of an agent of the Post, a man named Eustathios Bourtzes."

Metiga's face was unreadable, as was Uzun's, though the latter cast a glance at his brother.

"Early Tuesday morning, Bourtzes was found strangled not far from here," said Michael.

"Oh?" Uzun spoke in a thin voice. Michael expected more than a growl from him. "I think I hear something about it."

"No doubt you did. Many people have. And that's what I wanted to discuss with you." Michael turned towards Metiga. "It is known that you had a quarrel with Bourtzes."

Metiga's almond-shaped eyes became mere slits.

"It was about that affair last winter," Michael continued. "Bourtzes suspected that you might have brought on Tirakh Khan's attack."

The Patzinak managed a loose shrug. "But I did nothing," he said, flashing his teeth again. "He admitted that. I have witnesses."

"Witnesses—yes," said Michael, recalling the character of said witnesses. "But afterwards, were you and Bourtzes on good terms?" He fell silent: as if Metiga would tell him!

"Anyone can make mistake," said Metiga, spreading his hands. "I forgive him."

Michael arched an eyebrow. "That's an admirable Christian attitude... By the way, are you a Christian?"

"My uncle Kegen is and my mother, but I'm not. I receive the prayer, but I slide back."

Michael poured some water into his wine. "You mean that you were once made a catechumen, but that you're a backslider. Well, you have that trait in common with most of the human race."

A look of perplexity crossed Metiga's broad face, then vanished. Did he understand the jest?

"I'm heathen," Uzun said, laughing.

Michael glanced from Uzun's closed face back to his brother's. They were watching each other out of the corners of their eyes. Certainly, they were a wily pair.

But they didn't appear to be hiding anything, and innate cunning hardly made them guilty of Bourtzes's death.

"I'm sure you've done nothing wrong," Michael began again, "but where were you Monday night?"

Metiga bared his teeth and burst out laughing. "Here! At least I think so." He threw a questioning glance at Uzun.

The latter grinned. "Oh yes, we here all right. Drunk!"

Michael sighed inwardly. What had he expected? "Did you talk to anyone that night? Can you remember?"

Uzun frowned for a moment. "No, I can't. But the keeper—he vouch for us."

"I'm sure," said Michael. He'd have a word with the man later.

The Patzinaks exchanged glances again, poured themselves another cup apiece, and downed the wine in a single gulp. Uzun helped himself to more, but Metiga reached over and poked him in the ribs. "You better not, or you won't—"

Uzun set down his cup. "Well, let's go, hey?"

Michael could guess where they were headed, but he wouldn't let them go—not yet. He faced Uzun. "I gather you've been in the City for about a week. How do you like it?"

"Very good! Big buildings," he said, extending his hands. "And good food and drink, too."

"Of course," said Michael. Wine was certainly preferable to the fermented mare's milk that the nomads drank, and the variety of vegetables, grains, fish and meat in the City was certainly more appealing than the typical Patzinak fare of horse blood and millet.

106

Metiga stood up. "Isn't that enough? We go now."

"As you wish." Michael gazed at them reflectively. "I won't keep you from your…appointment any longer."

"Good," said Uzun, grinning broadly. "Perhaps we meet again, hey?"

Michael rose. "I'm sure we will." He watched as they crossed to the door, with long, bow-legged strides, the split skirts of their garments flapping against their hide breeches.

He would speak to the proprietor. He looked around and saw that the tavern was almost empty now. Only two chess players, huddled over their board, and several spectators remained. The proprietor and the help were washing cups.

Michael wondered how much his presence as a Court official had to do with the wine shop's dead atmosphere. True, it was long after the legal closing time, but most taverns stayed open late if they could get away with it.

"Sir?" Michael signaled the proprietor, who dropped his dishrag and plodded towards Michael's table, eyes downcast.

"Please have a seat." Michael indicated the chair opposite him.

The tavern-keeper sank into it.

"I'm not going to take action against you," said Michael. "In any case, that's not within my jurisdiction."

The proprietor's eyes widened in relief.

"I merely wanted to ask you about those two I was sitting with—the Patzinaks. Were they here Monday night?"

"Oh yes. Lately they've been here about every night."

"You mean for the past week or so?"

The tavern-keeper thought for a moment. "Yes."

"And before that?"

"The bigger, good-looking one came alone, almost every night."

Michael slumped his shoulders. Everything fit.

"Have they done something wrong?"

"I doubt it," said Michael, but told him about Bourtzes's murder.

The proprietor crossed himself. "I'd heard."

"Monday night he was checked in through a postern, during the second watch. Metiga has a possible motive for killing him."

The tavern-keeper thought for a moment. "I'm sure Metiga was here then. In fact, they both were, and *very* drunk when they arrived. It was not long after sundown."

"They told me they *thought* they were here Monday night...because they were in that state. How long did they stay?"

"Till morning."

Michael startled. "How can that be? Don't tell me they simply passed out under the table."

"No, sir. I put them to bed. I have a spare room in back, for just such cases."

Michael raised an eyebrow. "How charitable of you!"

The proprietor hunched over, pressing his arms close to his body. "Listen, I don't keep a disorderly house. I'm not a pimp!"

Michael stood up. "I'd like to see this room of yours."

"Ah—er—certainly!" The proprietor yanked himself to his feet, and, taking a candlestick from a nearby table, led

Michael to the back of the tavern.

Michael eyed a massive wooden door. "Is this it?"

"No, that leads outside."

"I see."

"The room is this way." The tavern-keeper turned left, escorting Michael down a hallway ending in another door. "Here." He threw it open and held up his candle.

Michael stepped into a squarish room containing two pallets covered with rough wool blankets. There was also a chamber pot, and a table equipped with a pottery basin, pitcher, and cups. He noticed a shuttered window in the far wall. "You're certain they were here the whole time?"

"I tell you—they were dead drunk when I put them to bed. And in the morning, when I came to rouse them, they were still asleep, and the window was latched."

"Which is not to say that it could not have been opened."

The tavern-keeper threw up his hands. "But I could see their condition!"

"What about the back door? Could they have gone out that way, then returned?"

"No. It's in plain view of the taproom, and it creaks."

"But the window?"

"Look, I know they were here all night."

"How can you be sure?"

"I watched them drop off to sleep, which didn't take long. Then I closed the door and went back to the taproom. Later, towards the end of the second watch of the night, as— er—my last customers were leaving, Metiga stumbled in. Ah—sorry, I hadn't closed yet," he added, cringing.

"What did he want?"

"He asked me to bring them a cup of wine to ward off the aches and pains in their heads."

"Did anyone else see him?"

The proprietor shrank. "Oh—I'm sure I could find men to vouch for him."

Exasperated, Michael let out his breath in a hiss. "Where was Uzun?"

"He was still asleep on his pallet when I brought in the wine."

"And you saw or heard nothing unusual, either here or outside?"

"No."

"Where did you go after you closed?"

He waved towards the staircase. "I live just upstairs. I heard nothing—all night."

Michael nodded. He didn't think the tavern-keeper was lying. He appeared to be the timid, servile type who would have been afraid to keep anything back.

But where did that leave Michael? Only with more questions.

Chapter 14

The next morning, before questioning anyone else, Michael attended Bourtzes's funeral in the Church of Hagia Eirene. Though he'd known the deceased only by sight and by his formidable reputation, he wished to pray for his soul.

Besides, funerals could sometimes provide insights into an investigation—though of course, Michael was not so naïve as to think that the murderer would appear and give himself away. Today, however, nothing had caught Michael's inquiring eye.

Surrounded by the clergy, the bier stood in front of the iconostasis, bathed in the light from the narrow windows in the dome. Bourtzes's widow and her two young sons—the elder looked around eight or nine—had already given Bourtzes the last kiss, and now the remaining mourners were filing up to the coffin. The service was almost over.

The pungent smell of incense pervaded the air. Michael peered through the clouds rising from many censers and watched Bourtzes's family as they retreated into the crowded nave. The lady, who had noble, olive-skinned features much like her husband's, looked sickly pale, and her eyes were swollen. If she did not cry now, certainly it was because she had already wept herself dry. They boys looked dazed, as though they couldn't comprehend what had happened.

Alas, when did youth ever understand death? Youth considered itself immortal, invulnerable. But what did the widow know about her husband's death. Lady Olympia might find out.

Michael began to search the crowd for her, but to no avail. He did see Acropolites approach the bier; most of the other high Court officials had already bade their farewells to the dead man.

Most of them… Michael now realized that he'd seen neither Psellus nor Blachernites.

What was wrong? Was the Emperor ill again? Had there been a crisis in the Palace? Or had the Logothete of the Dromos been *found out?*

Michael put his speculations aside, for the line was moving steadily; soon it would be his turn. Indeed, he found himself at the bier almost before he realized it. For the briefest of moments, he gazed upon Bourtzes.

He looked almost as handsome and imposing has he had in life. His dark hair and beard were well-combed, and he wore a white senatorial robe, while a jeweled gold whip—the insignia of his Court rank of *strator*—had been placed in his hand. He looked prepared to enter the next world giving a good account of his actions in this one.

Michael lowered his eyes in respect and bent to kiss Bourtzes's brow. He shuddered to find it cold. He felt the same at every funeral he had attended, including those—years apart—of his own parents. Death was an alien intrusion into life—an absurdity, even. Why should those he had known and loved—or, for that matter, not loved—be reduced to *this?*

With an inward groan, he moved away. The choir had begun the hymn that spoke for the departed: "As ye behold me lie before you all, speechless and bereft of breath, weep for me, O friends and brethren, O kinsfolk and acquaintance. For but yesterday I talked with you, but then there came upon me the dread hour of death."

Michael nodded. He had an intuition that he couldn't dismiss: the "dread hour of death" may have overtaken Bourtzes suddenly but not completely by surprise. If Michael only knew what the poor man had been doing that night...

Suddenly, the doors at the back creaked open, and a chill draft cut through the nave.

Michael stifled an impulse to spin around. Like the others in the crowd, he turned cautiously.

A familiar figure, a lanky man in a dark cloak, made his way through the parting throng. But instead of doing the expected—cutting into the line of mourners—he headed straight for Michael. "You're needed at the Palace now," said Psellus. "We have what we've been waiting for."

§

Minutes later, Psellus ushered Michael into Blachernites's office.

"Come in," said the wiry little man, and bolted the door behind them.

Michael bowed, then quickly surveyed the room. Psellus regained his seat—one of five chairs arranged in a semicircle. With him were the commander of the Varangians, and a thin, sandy-haired man whom Michael had never seen.

"Sit down," said the Logothete of the Dromos, and sank into his own chair, its back against his desk.

Michael sat next to Psellus and eyed the stranger.

"This is John Diogenes, an agent of ours," said the Logothete.

Diogenes nodded a greeting, then lowered his gaze. Above the line of his beard, his cheeks were a raw pink. His fingers, stiff from the cold, held a cup with difficulty. Despite his heavy wool tunic and breeches, he shivered.

"He rode in just this morning," said the Logothete. "He's been in Thessalonica since the spring—on routine business—and was stranded there during Tornicius's abortive revolt. He says that his stay was quite useful. He gained many insights into the politics of the provinces."

Michael frowned. "What has this to do with our present case?"

"You'll see. At our summons he finally set out for home, arriving in Philipoppolis about a fortnight ago. There he met Bourtzes—God rest his soul—who charged him with a great responsibility: Diogenes was to deliver his report to us."

The newcomer set down his cup and raised his gray eyes to the others. "He told me to wait until two days after his departure. Then I was to rush home with the document in question."

"What reason did he give you for these precautions?" Blachernites asked.

"He believed his life was in danger. He was being watched by hostile persons."

"There! You see?" The Logothete's gaze swept over the others.

The Akoluthos grunted.

"So, we know now that he was in danger," said Michael. "But isn't it curious that he was killed here in the

Capital...not in Philippopolis—that Sodom and Gomorrah—or on the road?"

Blachernites scowled. "Yes."

Michael turned to Diogenes. "What 'hostile persons' did he fear?"

The agent spread his hands. "He said the less he talked, the better. But I have an idea."

"It must be in the report," the Logothete said. "Let's read it together." He turned to pick up a rolled parchment from his desk, then smoothed it open on his lap. Skipping over the salutation and the recital of his titles, ranks, and honorifics, he began to read:

"'By the time you have this report, I will be either safely within the City, in which case you will find it superfluous, or else I will have departed on another mission, from which there is no return or recall...'" Blachernites faltered, swallowing awkwardly.

Michael exchanged glances with the others. They all crossed themselves, then lowered their eyes to the floor.

Finally, the Logothete drew a deep breath and continued. "'In either case, I hope that my observations will help you cleanse the western lands and indeed the whole Empire, of a most pernicious evil.'"

"'According to plan, I arrived in Philippopolis with a pack mule loaded with goods, in the guise of a 'harmless' official of the Imperial silk workshops of the Capital. I hoped that by selling off rather ordinary, or slightly defective garments to the provincials, I might become acquainted with the wealthy and influential of the area: not only government officials or army officers, but also well-to-do merchants or skilled craftsmen. I did indeed, and I also had many opportunities to observe the common people and the poor, since nobody connected me either with the Imperial Post or the local police...'"

Michael suppressed a smile and hoped that no one else noticed.

"'Alas, my findings, far from being encouraging, are positively alarming. The region is rife with heretics.'"

Psellus snorted. "We didn't need him to tell us that."

"Let's see what he's leading up to," the Logothete said, then continued reading:

"'First are the Armenians, who were originally settled here some years ago. Though they adhere to the Monophysite error preached by the church of their country, they participate in the life of the provinces and do not foment seditions. In fact, many of them serve in the army of the province Whatever they think of the Two Natures of Christ, most of them consider our presence better than the alternative. They would not wish to live in a rebel city or theme governed by lunatic sectarians.'"

"Again, that's no news," said Psellus, chewing on his mustache.

"That will do, Psellus. You're disgusting!" said Blachernites. His features twisted, as though he were in pain.

Michael felt a surge of nausea and forced it back. Psellus, he thought, liked to show off his erudition and be the center of attention. "Come now," he said. "Let's hear Bourtzes speak his piece."

"'But by far the largest and most powerful group of

heretics in Philippopolis is the Bogomils, who, though they subscribe to the same error of Manes as the Paulicians, are the product of local conditions. For the past seventy years or so, they've recruited their members from the local Slav peasantry—frustrated nationalists who consider themselves oppressed by the Empire. But recently the Bogomils have become influential in cities, and among the higher social strata, as well. Many well-to-do citizens belong to or support this sect—at least secretly. The most notable of these is the Mayor of Philipoppolis.'"

"Well!" The Logothete of the Dromos set the page on his lap. "Well!"

"Aren't we going to arrest him and—ah—put him to the question?" Psellus asked.

The Logothete waved him to silence. "We can't afford to be brutal." He picked up the parchment and turned it over. "Let's hear the rest of this. 'But one cannot say that the Bogomils keep to themselves. Indeed, membership in the sect is usually hard to prove because the Bogomils often pretend to be Orthodox and attend church to avert suspicion. They consider such dissembling justified: promises made to the 'devil' are worthless.'" Blachernites looked about to spit. "That corroborates everything we've ever heard about them. But back to the letter."

"'However, I think I beat them at their own game, at least for a while. I pretended to be one of them—a crypto-Bogomil, if you wish—and attended some of their meeting. It was thus that I learned of the involvement of the Mayor and others.

"'I also discovered something even more alarming than

this mass apostasy. Though the Bogomils, unlike the Paulicians, preach non-cooperation and passive resistance to authority, there is much talk among the Philippopolis group of secession from the Empire—specifically, of the creation of a Bogomil state extending from this city, on the south bank of the Marica river, all the way north to the Danube. Philipoppolis, of course, would be the capital and guardian of the new commonwealth.'"

The Logothete of the Dromos grasped the sides of the parchment, wrinkling them. "That's insane! How does a small segment of the population plan to gain control of a large area?"

"Remember," said Michael, "that particular territory is extremely hard to hold. As you know, we've been unable to expel rebellious Patzinaks from the area. If we've been able to control them to a certain extent, it's because they're a steppe people out of their element. On the other hand, our native, backwoods Bogomils are veritable mountain goats. What would happen if *they* instigated a revolt?"

"You have a point," said Psellus. "But the Bogomils aren't warlike."

"What if they plan to join with the Paulicians," asked Michael. "Or even the Patzinaks?"

"Wait!" put in the Logothete. "Let's see if Bourtzes enlightens us further: 'Still, how the Bogomils plan to accomplish this is anyone's guess. I could not find any evidence of the implementation of such a conspiracy, so I deem it wise to hold off arresting the Mayor and his confederates until we have positive proof...' That's just what I thought!"

John Diogenes, a practical man, surveyed the group. "But why not arrest and execute them all—for subscribing to a heresy that considers the Imperial authority the work of the devil. Certainly, that's tantamount to treason."

The Akoluthos clenched his fists. "Yes! Arrest them!"

The Logothete of the Dromos raised a restraining hand. "We'd look foolish—not to mention brutal, as I said. We need something to use against them."

Michael lowered his eyes. He abhorred violence and Draconian measures himself—as did many people, including the clergy. But was the Logothete truly reluctant to arrest the Mayor and his associates because he had no case against them, or did he have an ulterior motive?

Michael squeezed his eyes shut, as if that action could blot the thought from his mind.

Blachernites rustled the parchment insistently. "'Well, here's the conclusion of the report. 'Perhaps by the time of my return to the City, I will have found a solution. Or perhaps I will not return at all. I am currently being followed, and I fear my inn is under surveillance, though by whom or which faction, I don't know. In any case, I've discussed the situation with Naum Vladislavic, *Hypostrategos* of the theme, who will keep his eyes and ears wide open...'"

Michael straightened himself. "Why, that's Father Zosimas's brother!"

Lowering the page, Blachernites glanced at Michael. "Ahem! I gather you've caught up on that situation."

"I have—and they're lying!" Michael struggled to keep his voice even.

Blachernites raised his white eyebrows. "Oh?"

But Psellus nodded energetically. "I'm sure it's all nonsense. The State should do something to help out."

"I don't know what the State can do," said Michael, "but I plan to testify in Zosimas's favor." For the moment, he'd downplay his investigative role. After all, he was expected to spend all his time on Bourtzes's case.

"Um—we're not finished," said the Logothete. "Bourtzes has an interesting postscript. 'Now that I've mentioned the *Hypostrategos* of the theme, I recall something else: the Church wants to make his brother, Zosimas of the Studion, Bishop of Philippoppolis, the see being vacant. The people and the clergy of the theme support his candidacy, but the Bogomils are much opposed. A bishop from a popular local family would do much damage to their cause.'"

Michael jumped to his feet, recalling what he had heard from the Patriarch. "Well, there you have it! Why else would certain people be so eager to slander him?"

Chapter 15

Early in the afternoon, after a hurried and largely silent meal in one of the Palace dining rooms, Michael crossed the Augusteum to inform the Patriarch of what he had just learned about Zosimas. As usual, a servant ushered him upstairs, then left him at the Patriarch's oak door.

Michael knocked. "It's Michael Taronites."

"Come in."

Michael entered, and the Patriarch met him just inside. "Have you learned anything?"

"Your Holiness," Michael began, hurriedly kissing his hand. "I—"

The Patriarch put a fatherly arm around Michael's shoulders. "If you hadn't come now, I would have sent for you."

"What do you know?" Michael noticed a throbbing vein on the Patriarch's forehead.

"I'll tell you." The Patriarch indicated a chair in front of his desk, but he spoke of other matters. "So, we've interred Bourtzes, God rest his soul! Alas, I didn't go out to the cemetery. I have too many worries with this upcoming trial." He crossed himself, then sank into his desk chair. "I need some reassurance that we can clear our monk. Tell me what you've learned."

"But I thought you... Well, I've found out something that might help Father Zosimas."

"Oh?" The Patriarch looked up, his face brightening.

"I was called to the Palace during the funeral. An agent

of the Post had just brought in Bourtzes's missing report."

The Patriarch raised a heavy eyebrow.

"His dispatch confirms the fact that the clergy and people of Philippoppolis want Zosimas for their archbishop—just as you told me. But the local Bogomils do not."

"So, it's as we thought—the reason these accusations have arisen."

"I think so," said Michael. "Still, it's hard to believe that these accusers have a connection to the Bogomils of Philippoppolis, and I still need to find information to use against them."

"You haven't yet?"

"I will have by tomorrow, God willing." Michael dug his fingers into his palms. Everything took time—too much time. "But you wanted to tell me something?"

The Patriarch sighed. "Psellus, and—presumably—the Emperor have offered to stop the mouths of Zosimas's accusers and so eliminate the need for a trial. Have you heard anything about that?"

"This morning Psellus remarked that the State could help. I said I didn't see how."

"Good for you, and no thanks to the Palace. That would set a dangerous precedent, giving the State the right to meddle in Church affairs."

"It would."

"I trust we'll hear no more about it."

Michael cocked an eyebrow. "From the Court? Who can tell? But here's no way out of this situation but to prove our monk's innocence. Otherwise, these slanders will plague him—and us—forever."

"The Bogomils must be behind them," said the Patriarch.

"If only I can discover some Bogomil activity here in the City," said Michael, "and some connection with Philippopolis."

"That won't be easy," said the Patriarch. He inclined his head and thought for a moment. "Do you think that the Bogomils killed Bourtzes?"

"I don't know yet," said Michael. "But there must be some connection between the Bogomils's activities and Bourtzes's death—considering what he learned by spying on them. Er—this is between us, of course."

The Patriarch cleared his throat. "Of course!"

"Bourtzes learned that the Bogomil heresy is flourishing in Philippopolis. It's no longer the faith only of peasants. Many craftsmen, merchants, public officials and nobles have also embraced it."

"God help us." The Patriarch rested his head in his hands.

Only when he looked up again, did Michael speak. "So, if a connection exists between the Bogomils of Philippopolis and those in the City, and between Bourtzes's murder and the campaign against Zosimas, I intend to find it."

Chapter 16

Michael deemed it wise to learn more about the history of Bogomilism and related heresies, so the next hour found him beneath the high, vaulted ceiling of the Patriarchal library. The Great Chartophylax—the Librarian or Keeper of the Documents—assigned an assistant to him, a youthful sub deacon named Cyril.

He settled Michael at a table beneath some arched windows and supplied him with a pen, ink, and parchment scraps. These, Michael noticed, were actually the reverse sides of old letters, or the rough drafts of sermons.

With his back to the windows, he sat down, enjoying the warmth of the pale sunlight. Moments later, Cyril brought him an armload of books and scrolls gleaned from the library's cabinets and pigeonholes. "This is most of what we have on the Manicheans, Paulicians, and Bogomils," he said, plunking them on the table and raising a puff of dust.

Michael selected a book on the Manicheans.

"Did you know," Cyril began, "that the beginning of the Creed refutes both the Manicheans and the Gnostics? 'I believe in one God, the Father Almighty, Maker of heaven and earth, and of all things visible and invisible.'"

"Yes, I can see that."

"You ought to read St. Irenaeus of Lyons on the Gnostics as well."

"Thank you, but I have my hands full."

"Then I'll tell you about them in short: they believed that the world was created not by God, but by the demiurge."

"What we'd call the devil," Michael concluded.

Michael undid the clasps on his book and opened it, while Cyril examined another volume.

Manes, Michael read, had begun his preaching in Persia, some seventy years before the reign of Constantine the Great. Manes's followers, known from the first as Manicheans, were considered heretics by both the Christians and the Zoroastrians, though they were quite close to the latter in teaching. In fact, just as the prophet Zoroaster had taught that the world was ruled by two equal but opposite deities—the holy spirit and the evil spirit, which were both created by the supreme god Ahura Mazda—so did Manes hold that the world was governed by the forces of Light and Darkness. Light he identified with the spirit and heavenly beings, Darkness with the physical and the material. Man was a combination of both—in which was his tragedy—but Jesus Christ, the God of Light's greatest messenger, was a completely spiritual being who only appeared to be a man. He alone could rescue the Light held captive in man's brutal physical nature.

Michael paused; how strange!

Man, being a combination of Light and Darkness, could not wholly be saved. Only the spiritual part of his nature was worthy of salvation, and the goal of his existence was the return of the Light to its source—the good God, the Light. Thus, the ideal life was one which avoided all contact with the physical world.

However, since not everyone could manage such austerity, only the Elect were required to fulfill the

Manichean commandment perfectly: they could not drink wine, marry, or engage in any manual labor. The ordinary believers, called Hearers, were forbidden to eat meat because some small fragment of the Light resided in animal flesh. These faithful were also enjoined to fast at certain times, but they could employ themselves in any manner, except, perhaps, as soldiers. They were even permitted to marry, though fornication and random sexual encounters were considered much less depraved than matrimony.

This, Michael thought, was what everyone said about the Bogomils. He nudged Cyril and whispered, "Do you find that all dualists adhere to this manner of thought?"

"Definitely."

Michael closed the book and fastened the clasps, then reached for another volume. It was a slender work, written perhaps fifty years ago by the Bulgarian priest Cosmas, and was considered the definitive anti-Bogomil polemic.

"In the days of the Orthodox Tsar Peter, there lived in the land of Bulgaria a priest called Bogumil, who in reality was not loved by God."

Michael managed a sick smile. There had been no Bulgarian kingdom—or tsardom—for over thirty years—not since Emperor Basil II, appropriately called the Bulgar-Slayer, had blinded 14,000 Bulgarian captives, leaving one in each hundred with a single eye so that they could guide the remaining ninety-nine back to their king. The grisly spectacle made Samuel, the last Tsar of Bulgarian, collapse with a fatal apoplexy.

Now Michael re-read Cosmas's opening sentence in bewilderment, then looked at the translator's marginal

126

note. Cosmas had availed himself of what was a glorious pun in Slavonic: Bogumil, the heretic's name, meant "loved of God," or "dear to God," whereas Cosmas insisted that he was not loved of God—"Bogu *ne* mil."

Certainly not. Michael read further in Cosmas's account of Bogomil doctrines. They appeared to be a warmed-over mishmash of Manichean beliefs and—Michael suspected—local peasant customs. According to the sect's teachings, everything material was created by the devil, and the miracles of the New Testament were merely allegories, for God would never touch devil-created matter. Thus, the Old Testament was inspired by the devil because it credited the good God with the creation of the world.

Cyril was looking over Michael's shoulder. "They consider the villains of the Old Testament heroes—Cain, the Sodomites, the Egyptians..."

"I can grasp the idea."

Michael continued reading. According to Cosmas, the Bogomils accepted the four Gospels and the Acts of the Apostles. Their rule of prayer consisted of reading these, as well as repeating the Lord's prayer four times daily and four times nightly. They treated the Mother of God with appalling disrespect and rejected all rites of the Church because they made use of the material. They did not venerate icons, and they detested the Cross both as a material object and an instrument of torture.

The Bogomils neither ate meat nor drank wine. They were discouraged to marry, forbidden to shed blood, and positively enjoined to disobey authority. "They denounce the wealthy, loath the Tsar, ridicule the elders, condemn the nobles," Cosmas stated. Still, they pretended to be Orthodox and played the part of law-abiding citizens. "Sheep," Cosmas called them—hypocritical sheep.

Still, though Cosmas's description of the heresy was quite detailed and matter-of-fact, it was not much help to someone trying to hunt down members of the sect.

Nor had Cosmas pronounced the last word on the Bogomils. The scribe and translator had added more notes of his own in the margins: the Bogomils, like the Manicheans, had two classes of believers, the ordinary and the Elect, or Perfect. It was these latter who did not eat meat or other animal foods, drink wine, or marry; if the world belongs to the devil, they concluded, have nothing to do with it. But the less strict Bogomils often went to the opposite extreme: they ate and drank what they pleased, married, and often engaged in the most frightful licentiousness. If you already belonged to the devil, they reasoned, one more sin won't hurt you.

Michael frowned. What drove a person to believe that the devil had created the world? The weight of constant misfortune, perhaps, or simple human perversity? He wasn't cynical enough—yet—to believe that people were merely seeking an excuse to sin.

Cosmas, for his part, did not attempt to answer *why* the Bogomils believed as they did, though he tried to explain the sect's growing popularity. The Orthodox themselves were to blame, he said, because they abandoned their wives and children, served their masters poorly, while their clergy lived in luxury and their rulers in debauchery. So, by setting a deplorable example and behaving as though the devil indeed ruled the world, they encouraged those of little faith to go even further in their sins.

How true! Michael thought. The Court was rife with plots and intrigues, and the Emperor, who claimed to be God's Vice-Regent, amused himself with a young mistress and mocking buffoons like Saponas.

Saponas! What did he have to do with Bourtzes—and with Zosimas?

If Saponas was a Bogomil, he was clearly no moralist. But some Bogomil converts, perhaps the well-to-do citizens of Philippopolis, must be moralists with a vengeance, moralists who had grown disgusted with the Empire's wickedness.

Once Michael had exhausted Cosmas's knowledge, he put the book aside. Now the light from the windows was dimmer. It was past time for him to continue his questioning. He must speak with Tripsychos, Bourtzes's rival in love, with that odious shopkeeper, Peter of Serrhes, with those evil tongues at the Studion.

But Cyril was not about to let him go. He raised one hand to restrain Michael, and pushed an open book towards him with the other. Its musty scent seeped into Michael's nostrils. "You've forgotten the Paulicians," he said.

At first the book told Michael nothing he didn't know. The Bogomils were in fact an offshoot of the Paulician sect, many of whose members had been forcibly resettled from Armenia and Eastern Anatolia to Macedonia and Thrace. Here they could be of some use to the Empire, for their prowess in battle helped keep marauding barbarians at bay. Indeed, the chief difference between the Bogomils and the

Paulicians was their attitude towards war.

Still, as Michael read on, he found much that was new to him. John of Otzun, an Armenian bishop, accused the Paulicians of such abominations as worshipping the sun and the demons of the air, exposing their dead on rooftops, and mixing the blood of babies with their communion food.

Michael gulped. Exactly what Psellus had said this morning! The fact had been revolting then, but now Michael's noon meal of sausage and vegetables cooked in olive oil weighed on his stomach like a stone colossus.

He skimmed a few more pages, then stopped, intrigued. The Paulicians had first come upon the Imperial scene some three centuries ago. Soon afterwards, they established a free state beyond the Empire's frontier. It went without saying that their "government" had the backing of the neighboring Muslim emirs, to whom they sold captives from the Empire as slaves.

The Paulicians' life was one of frequent raids into Imperial territory, promiscuity, illegitimacy, incest, and purges in which one faction tried to establish true equality by massacring all its opponents.

And for a time, the influence of the Paulicians was as great as their menace: several high-ranking officials of the Empire defected to them.

Then, less than two hundred years ago, Emperor Basil I led an army against the seat of the Paulician community at Tephrike, hoping to destroy it utterly. Instead, he nearly died in the attempt, and only the heroism of certain Armenian peasants enabled him to retreat from the fury of the heretics. Of these Armenians, the best known was the father of the then future Emperor Romanus Lecapenus.

Michael read on: undaunted, the Paulicians continued their destructive raids into the heart of Anatolia. Two years after the failed campaign, Emperor Basil sent another army against them. This time the Imperial troops had better luck. As the Paulicians, weighted down with copious booty, made a slow march homeward, a certain Gregory of Argaoun, a deserter from the heretic army, directed the Imperials to their campsite. The Paulicians soon found themselves surrounded—at which time Pulades, a captive buffoon, stabbed their leader Chrysocheir, "the Golden Hand."

Strange, thought Michael. For all their democratic sentiments, they couldn't manage without a leader.

Immediately following the death of Chrysocheir, the Paulician community disbanded, and when the Imperial troops pushed through to Tephrike, they found it deserted. Thus, the heretics' state crumbled into dust, while those who had betrayed it were covered with honor and glory.

Michael observed that at this point the scribe had inserted a marginal note: "The descendants of Gregory of Argaoun now play a prominent part in Court life, though they hold that their place of origin is not the disreputable Paulician settlement of Argaoun, but the city of Raban, far to the south. The family has since changed its name to Syropoulos."

Michael startled. *Syropoulos!* He reached for his pen and a parchment scrap. So that was what ailed the man.

As Michael rustled the parchments, Cyril looked up from his book. "Well, sir, I see you've found something enlightening."

"Indeed," said Michael. "I have."

Chapter 17

Olympia had attended Bourtzes's funeral, and afterwards, she and her eunuchs accompanied the mourners to a cemetery outside the walls, near the Adrianople Road. A touch of irony, that! She was aware that Bourtzes had taken this route on the fateful night he returned to Constantinople.

Later she returned with the mourners to Bourtzes's house for the funeral meal. She had made certain that her servants brought gifts of sweet wine, Russian caviar, and honey cake. She wished to make a kindly gesture, though it was poor consolation for a woman who had just lost her husband.

After the meal, Olympia, acting on her teacher's orders, persuaded the family's many kinsfolk and friends to leave her alone with the widow for the night.

"Everybody out," she said. "Come back in the morning." With the cooperation of the household servants, she believed she could manage things best.

Indeed, the guests departed by dusk, when shadows had gathered in the corners of the dining room.

"It's time you got some rest," said Olympia, placing a hand on the widow Marina's shoulder.

The latter turned a splotchy, tear-stained face to Olympia. "Can you take me upstairs?"

"Of course." Olympia slipped the strap of her medical bag over one arm and grasped her additional burden, a bulky cloth-wrapped package, by the twine that bound it. With her free hand, she took Marina's elbow and helped her up the broad marble staircase.

When they reached the second floor, Marina directed her to a sitting room intended for the use of the family only. Its small-paned windows looked out on the roofs and domes of the hillside, where the Column of Marcian was limned against a darkening, red-streaked sky.

Olympia directed the widow to a curved-backed couch. "You can stretch out there."

"I can sit," said Marina. And did so, stiffly planting her feet on the floor.

Olympia drew up a chair. Marina clasped her hands in her lap and would not speak.

Olympia did not know what to say. Though she felt great pity for Marina, she hadn't come here simply on her teacher's instructions, or on an errand of mercy. She hoped to learn something more about Bourtzes's life...and death. In fact, she had seen Michael leave the funeral with Psellus. Had they learned something new?

Olympia noticed that the widow's swarthy skin looked sickly pale beneath reddish splotches. The shadows around her reddened eyes were almost the shade of the black kerchief wound tightly over her head.

Olympia felt her throat tighten. The poor woman was distraught from weeping. Wouldn't it be cruel and unfeeling to question her now?

But perhaps she'd feel better if she talked.

Then Olympia felt a draft. A manservant, a eunuch had entered, closing the door behind him. He padded across the patterned carpet to the brazier. "Sir," she asked, as he stirred the charcoal fire, "could you bring us some wine and warm water, and some food?"

Marina startled, as though she had just returned to the world of the living. "You don't have to, Damian. I'm not hungry."

That did it. Now Olympia would assume the role of doctor. "Do so anyway," she said, rising. "She needs it."

She gave Marina a stern look. "I was watching you during the meal. You hardly ate a thing. Indeed, have you eaten or slept at all for the past two days?"

Marina bowed her head. "No, but what does it matter?"

Olympia exchanged glances with Damian, who still looked uncertain. "Please! Go quickly!"

Once he'd left the room, Olympia loosened her own head covering. She sat down beside Marina and hugged her strongly. The widow shuddered, then rested her head on Olympia's shoulder and was still.

"I know you don't care for yourself," said Olympia. "But you have two small boys who need you. You can't give up."

Marina's slender body began to shake.

"And then there's your husband—may God rest his soul. The best way to honor his memory is to fight the good fight."

"But I—"

"I know," said Olympia, though she was unsure what Marina would say. "But first of all, you need to rest, to recover your strength."

So, Marina did not protest when Olympia placed her head on a cushion, removed her soft leather shoes, and arranged more pillows under her feet. Last of all she positioned a small, ivory-inlaid table directly in front of the couch. If only Damian came back soon!

Olympia walked over to the windows and looked out, past the houses, towards the blackening waters of the Propontis. Night was settling in.

"I might as well close the curtains," she said, grasping a panel of heavy silk and pulling it across a window. The rings made a harsh sound as they scraped across the metal rod.

"You don't have to do that." Marina's voice cracked with exhaustion. "Damian will."

"It's all right." Olympia drew the remaining curtain. Then, to her relief, she heard footsteps on the staircase. When she turned, Damian was waiting in the doorway, holding a tray.

"Thank you," said Olympia. "You can set it on the table. And you may go now."

As the door shut behind him, Olympia turned her attention to the tray. It held ewers of wine and warm water and a small vessel of honey. So far so good.

There was also a plate of sliced bread, a block of goat cheese, a dish of olive oil, and a bowl containing a small mound of black caviar—the kind she had brought.

"Now, as a physician, I'm going to insist that you eat." She poured equal parts wine and water into two goblets, adding a generous spoonful of honey to each. "That done, she heaped food onto a reddish pottery plate and extended her hand to Marina. "So, you'd better sit up."

Marina smoothed her skirts and took a few desultory sips of wine before she set down the cup with a resounding clunk. She buried her face in her hands. "I don't know who could have wanted him dead!"

Olympia slipped and arm around her. Once more her throat closed up. "It doesn't make sense, does it?"

"He was a good man. Nobody had any cause to hate him."

But Olympia thought that the good always had enemies—namely the wicked.

"Surely he will inherit the Heavenly Kingdom," said Marina. "Don't you think so?"

"I think we can believe that."

Gradually the tremors racking Marina's shoulders subsided. She pulled away and sat up. Tears continued to stream down her face.

Olympia offered her a plain handkerchief. "However, though we should all pray for the repose of his soul, some of us have practical concerns as well. The Palace wants to find the person responsible for his death so that he doesn't perpetrate more such abominations." Now she was no longer speaking as a doctor.

Marina gave her eyes a final dab, then set her handkerchief aside. "But there's nothing I can tell you. I have no idea—"

"You may know more than you think you do."

"But he never discussed his work with me, or not much."

Olympia had expected that. Still, satisfied that Marina seemed ready to talk, she picked up her cup and returned to her seat. "Considering what he did, that's as it should be," she said.

"Yes. He always said his work was highly secret."

"But he might have given you some general idea of his

assignments."

"He did." Marina pensively dipped a piece of bread into the olive oil.

"He said he was investigating the heretics in Philippopolis," she said. "And last summer, he said he was going to foil Tornicius. It was only later that I found out that he impersonated a soldier in Tornicius's army. When I think of the risks he took—" She reached for her handkerchief again.

Olympia set down her cup. "I understand. But, do you recall: before he set out for Philippopolis did he seem especially worried or preoccupied?"

"He was always like that. For as long as I can remember, I had the feeling that there was more going through his mind than he let on."

"Ah—no doubt that's common in his line of work." But Olympia had no such impression of Michael. But then, he was new to the Post.

"I suppose so, but—" Marina clenched her handkerchief, then let it drop in her lap. "I didn't know he was in so much danger—"

Olympia's fair eyebrows drew together. "I wonder if he knew himself." She felt a dangerous moment approaching.

"I never had a chance to say goodbye to him. I—" Marina's mouth tensed as she stifled a sob, then looked away.

Olympia returned to the couch and sat down next to her again, with Marina's head on her shoulder. The widow's tears soaked through Olympia's garment, straight to her skin. Olympia hugged her close.

For some time, neither spoke. Gradually the tension ebbed from Marina's shoulders, and she moved away, dabbing at her eyes and blowing her nose loudly. "Oh—excuse me!"

"It's all right." Olympia refilled Marina's cup and held it to her lips. "Drink this at least. You'll feel better." Getting the lady to eat more was probably too much to hope for.

When Marina had finished the wine, Olympia put the cup aside, then regarded her in silence. She appeared calmer, though her eyes were still red.

Now, thought Olympia, it might be possible to talk seriously. But she must proceed cautiously. "If you feel like talking, I have some questions for you. If not, I can come back another day."

"As you wish. I'm afraid I haven't been much help."

"The authorities are still trying to find the person who killed your husband. Now, there's a possibility that his death may have had nothing to do with his mission, but instead..." Olympia felt awkward bringing up such a sensitive matter.

"Instead what?" Marina's voice was flat, as if she didn't know what Olympia was implying.

"There could have been some personal rivalry between him and another man. Does the name Gregory Tripsychos mean anything to you?"

Olympia saw a flicker of recognition in her eyes.

"Why—yes. He was a suitor of mine. But that was over ten years ago, before—He couldn't possibly—"

"Are you aware that last spring he and your husband had a...rather vocal altercation in the halls of the Post."

Marina startled. "Really? Why?"

"I believe it was over something rather trivial. The Logothete of the Dromos received Bourtzes first and obliged Tripsychos to wait in the hall."

"I had no idea." Her red-streaked eyes regarded Olympia frankly.

"I see," said Olympia. "But, can you tell me about your acquaintance with Tripsychos?"

"I never so much as spoke to him, though I knew who he was. We saw each other in the atrium of the church. He used to sit by the fountain. And then, once or twice, he was invited to dinner at the family home on some feast day. I caught only a glimpse of him—even though I knew he'd asked my father for my hand—or sent someone else to."

"Of course." Olympia suppressed a snort of derision. Of course, it happened that way! The men and women would have dined apart, and a single man would have been kept far away from all unmarried girls. "Now, I presume you—er—met your husband in the same way?"

"Yes. Both men asked my father for my hand, and he decided."

Olympia cleared her throat. So much for marriage among us! Though parents usually meant well, and—she had to admit—chaperones were advisable in most cases, it was absurd to keep a girl from speaking with the man she might spend the rest of her life with. *That* was not what impaired one's virginity.

Nevertheless, she kept her opinions to herself. "So, how did your father arrive at his choice?"

"Tripsychos was rather poor."

Olympia nodded. Again, there was nothing surprising here. Wealth was usually the deciding factor. Still, she could see the good sense in choosing a man of means for one's daughter—though she hoped she never found herself in Marina's position.

"Do you think that your rejected suitor has harbored a grudge?"

Marina managed a weak smile. "I don't know. I haven't seen him for ten years."

"No?"

Marina's eyes widened. "No! I may have seen him in a public place. That's all."

"He hasn't ever tried to contact you? Not recently?"

"Why no!"

"I see," said Olympia. She could see that Marina was telling the truth. The poor woman was too naïve to dissemble. And so far she had revealed nothing that would lead Olympia—and Michael—to the killer.

Now she tried another approach. "Can you tell me about your husband's family? I thought that the Bourtzes were a military family with lands in the Anatolic theme."

"They are. But generations ago there was a quarrel. Afterwards…his great-grandfather came to the Capital and entered the civil service."

"Does this antagonism still exist?"

"Not that I know of. But the two branches of the family have little to do with each other."

"Oh." Olympia slumped her shoulders. She was weary and had to force herself to get up. "Forgive me for keeping you so long. If you'd like to retire now, I'll summon your maid. I can spend the night here, in this room, in case you need anything."

"All right."

Olympia paused, studying Marina's tear-stained face. "Tomorrow your family can return. But send for me in any case—if you need anything or simply if you want some company." She spoke as a physician, as one whose first duty, along with healing, was to show compassion.

Before she turned to go, Olympia retrieved her bag, which she'd left by her chair, and extracted a small metal vial. "My master sent you something to help you sleep tonight." She shook several drops into a cup of water and stirred it. The sweetish, heavy fumes of a poppy decoction hung in the air.

Then Olympia noticed the package she'd also left by her seat; why, she'd almost forgotten it! "I brought the...effects found with your husband, and a list. Let's go through them to make certain that nothing's missing."

Marina rose shakily. "All right. But most of them I won't keep. I'll summon the deacons and have them distribute his clothing to the poor. And now I'll sort through all his things in the house. There's no point in hoarding them."

"That's a wise decision," said Olympia, "but now..." She set the bundle on the couch and untied the cords. Then, as Marina unwrapped it the rest of the way and began poking through the contents, Olympia picked up the enclosed list. "'Wool cap and cloak,'" she read, "'wool tunic and hose, cotton undertunic and drawers, leather boots and belt, a belt pouch containing a few coppers.' His signet ring was buried with him—there's a note of that here."

Marina nodded, then continued rummaging through the clothing.

"'Two complete changes of clothes—similar to the above,'" Olympia continued. "'These were found in his saddle bags, as was one long dress tunic of maroon wool. Also, a comb and a cake of soap. The official mail that he carried, as well as his bow, bow case, and a quiver containing thirty-five arrows, were repossessed by the Post.'" But Michael had been convinced that something—he knew not what—was missing from the list.

Marina began to refold the garments carefully. "Everything's here that should be—but wait!" Her pencil-line eyebrows drew together. "Something's missing. Where's his cross?"

"Wasn't it buried with him?"

"No! Or at least you made no note of it, as you did with his ring."

Chapter 18

Michael was about to leave the Patriarchate when someone started banging on the back door. A servant opened it with trembling hands, and a strapping Varangian Guard, the cause of the racket, strode in. "So, there you are, Taronites! We have something for you."

"Let's go then."

Thick dusk had descended on the City. Since the Brazen Gates were now closed, they entered the Palace through a guarded postern.

Their destination was the headquarters of the Varangian guard. Michael choked back a lump of dread. Would he have to admit his lack of progress to the commander?

They found the Akoluthos at his desk, writing on a parchment. Light from a bronze oil lamp shone on his silver-blond hair.

He was not alone; a tall, well-proportioned man sat to one side, his dark curly head bowed, his hands folded in his lap. Michael found him vaguely familiar.

"Sir?" asked the Varangian who accompanied Michael.

The Akolouthos looked up and turned his hard, iron-gray gaze to Michael. "We've finally located this very elusive gentleman," he said, nodding towards his visitor. "We've already questioned him, but we're certain you'll have something to ask him yourself. This is Gregory Tripsychos."

Tripsychos looked up. "Good evening."

"The same to you," said Michael. "I—ah—didn't quite recognize you. Your name is more familiar to me than your face." And what a face! Austere yet comely, it belonged on an icon of St. Theodore Stratilates, or another soldier saint.

Tripsychos winced. "I'm sure you know—"

Michael addressed the Akoluthos. "I trust that you questioned him politely."

"Of course! But he's told us nothing we didn't know."

Michael turned back to Tripsychos. "Your Honor..." The man's hair and beard looked slightly damp. He was still unwell then.

"You've been hard to reach lately." Michael eyed the left sleeve of Tripsychos's well-fitted tunic. It bulged around the upper arm; there must be a bandage underneath. "Is your wound still bothering you?"

Tripsychos dipped his head. "Yes. I haven't been coming in every day."

"Perhaps you should stay in bed—or be admitted to the hospital."

Tripsychos's eyes, large and very dark, met Michael's. "I don't like to neglect my duties. The hurt's getting better, anyway. And I go to the hospital for treatment. Just his morning I had my dressing changed."

"You go to St. John's Hospital?"

"Yes. I live nearby."

"Were you there Monday night? And at what time?"

"I don't recall exactly—during the second watch of the night."

Michael nodded. The man's story matched that of his servants, which did not necessarily make it true. But it was quite convenient, for no one knew the exact time of Bourtzes's death.

"Your doctors will vouch for your condition, I presume."

"Of course."

"Exactly when were you wounded?"

"Last Thursday. I lost a lot of blood."

Michael smiled ruefully. "A man in your condition could not have assaulted Bourtzes singlehandedly."

"But I didn't—" said Trispsychos. A pained expression crossed his face.

"Of course you didn't." Michael wanted to believe him. He found the man's silent, melancholy disposition sympathetic.

Tripsychos slumped his shoulders in relief, or perhaps in weariness.

"I'm sorry, but we're not quite finished here," said Michael.

"Oh?"

"Is there anyone who can vouch for you besides your servants?"

"No. I'm a widower, and if I had a wife, you wouldn't believe her testimony."

"I'm sorry." Michael lowered his eyes. Loss was always painful—as well he knew. But was he too sensitive to others' feelings, and to his own, to be a good interrogator? "Forgive me. When did...?"

"Five years ago. My wife died in childbirth. And my little girl."

"I'm so sorry." Michael could think of nothing else to say. Still, he must be circumspect. What if Tripsychos had recovered from his grief and rekindled his passion for Bourtzes's wife? "How well did you know Bourtzes?"

"Not well, really. He was far above me, and he was often out of town, in any case."

"But last spring you quarreled with him in public." Michael indicated the Akoluthos. "This man has witnesses."

"I won't deny it. I lost control of myself."

When else had the man lost control? "What about Bourtzes's wife?" Michael inquired. "You paid court to her at one time."

Tripsychos blinked, and Michael regretted asking him such a hard question.

"I did. But she—or rather her father—refused me."

Now it was Michael's turn to flinch. How would Olympia's father deal with *him,* if he were in a similar position? And what would he do, if she were "given" to another?

At last, he spoke. "Have you spoken with her since that time?"

"No."

"Not even while Bourtzes was away on assignment? Not even recently?"

Tripsychos squared his shoulders; he understood. "No! That happened so long ago. I told the Akoluthos."

"True." Michael knit his brows in frustration. "That's enough for tonight," he said. "Dismissed."

Enough for tonight, perhaps, but not for long.

§

After leaving the commander's office, Michael headed deeper into the Palace compound. He intended to stop by his own office to see if he'd received any messaged or report.

A canopy of stars hung high over the hillside. The night

was chilly, and a gust of icy wind blew into his face. He huddled his beard into his cloak but pressed on, past a grove of shifting trees, black and formless.

Then he heard the rustle of dry leaves. A twig snapped behind him, and his stomach clenched.

Heart pounding, he dashed ahead. The while walls of the Pavilion of the Pearl, the Augusta's summer residence, loomed before him. Beyond was a well-lit avenue. Once there in the lanterns' glow, he drew a deep breath. No one would dare attack him here.

Further on, a blaze of light crowned the golden dome of the Great Chrysotriclinium. Windows glowed in the office wing behind it—Michael's destination.

At the nearest entrance, the night guard recognized him and waved him in. "You too!"

Michael wondered who else was here.

Once in the corridor, Michael saw light beneath the Logothete's door. But Michael wouldn't question him yet. He still felt awkward about suspecting his own boss.

Michael mounted the stairs to his office, where, according to regulations, the door was left open. He went in and fumbled on his desk for a taper, then retreated into the corridor to light it from a wall sconce.

He applied the flame to the wick of the painted clay lamp on his desk, and a dust-flecked glow flooded the windowless cubicle. It revealed a single sheet of parchment—an invitation to a reception tomorrow night, in the Emperor's apartments.

Well! he wondered. Why had he been included?

His spirits sank when he arrived at the most likely

conclusion: the Emperor wanted a report on Bourtzes's case. Still, Michael doubted that the frivolous Monomachus would spoil a social occasion with State business.

In any case, Michael would have to go, though he felt doubly foolish: he had neither found Bourtzes's murderer nor cleared Father Zosimas.

Somehow, he would remedy that. Tomorrow he'd make time to watch the shop of Peter of Serrhes, and he would speak to Zosimas as well.

Satisfied, he folded the invitation and stuffed it into his belt pouch. Then, still mindful of the thing that had stalked him in the trees, he extinguished the lamp and left.

Chapter 19

Though Friday morning dawned chill and rainy, Michael set out early, eager to reach the Palace as soon as the Brazen Gates opened. His first task was to consult Syropoulos about his Paulician ancestors. Then he would tend to his business out in the City.

As he rode down the Mese, an alarm sounded in his mind. Last night, after he'd left the Palace, no one pursued him. But earlier someone had stalked him on the Palace grounds. And the night before, when he'd been searching taverns, he was certain someone was following him. The matter was far from settled. He should assume that he was being watched.

Once inside the Palace, he headed for the Imperial offices, but both the Emperor's portals and Syropoulos's door were closed. No matter; the *Kanikleios* might still be in.

"Your Excellency?" Michael called, knocking repeatedly. No one answered or stirred inside. He might as well come back another time.

On his way out, he stopped a Varangian guard. "Did Syropoulos come in today?"

"No."

"Is he ill?"

The rangy fellow merely shrugged.

§

It was still early, not yet the third hour, when Michael rode home to change clothes. He donned a brief, unadorned wool tunic and a cloak of coarse wool, that he'd often worn when he lived on his estates in the East. And just to make certain he wouldn't be associated with the Post, he removed his signet ring and put it in his belt pouch. Last of all he attached his sheath and knife to his belt. He could hide it under his cloak.

The rain had stopped, and the clouds were lifting when he set out on foot to find Peter of Serrhes's grocery. It was not far from Michael's house: up one narrow street and north on another. Along the way, the buildings looked respectable enough: one- or two-story houses and large stone apartment blocks with shops on the ground floor. Only the dark maw of an occasional alleyway made him uneasy.

Was somebody actually following him? He turned a corner, following the directions a militiaman had given him, and sighted Peter's house, three stories with a gabled tile roof. It stood at the end of the block, across the street.

As Michael quickened his step, fat droplets from the earlier rain plopped from a balcony onto his shoulder. First these caught his attention, and then something else did: a sound fainter than a whisper, a movement quicker than the blinking of an eye.

He threw himself against the wall of the house and dropped to his knees. Something whined overhead and slammed into the stone not two feet above him. He shut his eyes, then forced himself to open them again.

He crawled forward, and an arrow clattered to the pavement just in front of him. It must have come from the other side of the street, from a window or rooftop.

On his feet again, stooped like a hunchback, he ran for

the nearest alley, praying that it was not a trap. He dove in—and not a moment too soon: another shaft hissed by him, thudding into the wall of a wooden house.

Mother of God, save me! Breathing raggedly, he moved down the alley, keeping his back against the nearest house. Had the assault stopped? He freed his arms from his cloak and grasped the hilt of his dagger, then made his way deeper in.

No new ambush awaited him—thank God! At least not yet.

Only when his heart stopped pounding and his breathing slowed did he notice the stink of rotten vegetables and stale urine. Now he shrank from the wall in disgust, casting a quick glance backwards. He was not about to retrace his steps but wouldn't give up, either. He'd find another way to Peter's store.

He sheathed his knife and followed the alley to a street broader than the one he'd been on. After peering out and looking both ways, he headed north, watching the houses on the far side and keeping his distance from those on his own. When he'd gone two blocks further than Peter's store, he drew his dagger and turned into another murky alley. He pulled back at the sound of a scuffle.

But when his eyes reaccustomed themselves to the dark, he saw no cause for alarm—only a pair of snarling cats fighting a bevy of rats. He kicked a stone at the latter and watched in satisfaction as they scurried off. A cold sweat ran down his back.

When he reached the far end of the alley, he peered out and surveyed the scene. There was no one on the rooftops.

All the upper-story windows were shuttered. Was it safe?

He sheathed his dagger again and headed back towards the tall house with the gabled roof. With an involuntary shudder, he wondered if the archer was waiting for him at the grocery.

Not very likely! And perhaps the sniper had no connection with Peter. Michael had been followed for the past two nights, so perhaps a certain someone didn't want him nosing around anywhere.

He shrugged, if only to convince himself to be calm. Then, pulling his cloak forward over the dagger at his belt, he crossed the cobbled street.

The grocery's rough-planked, unpainted door gave a loud creak as he opened it, and the shop's interior was in no better condition. Its walls, perhaps once closer to white, were now gray. And though the day was dismal, no lamps or candles burned. The owner must be frugal, if not downright stingy.

No one attended the counter either, though a handbell had been left there. So where was the serpent-tongued slanderer?

Michael waited, breathing in the familiar smells of salt fish and goat cheese. After a few moments, he heard voices from an adjacent room—the grocer's living quarters, no doubt. He noticed a door behind the counter.

No one opened it.

"Hello?" Michael said, and rang the bell.

That brought results. The door opened promptly, and a beardless youth, ambled in, closing it behind him. Though he was only of average height, he had two outstanding features: longish chestnut hair and large eyes of nearly the same color. A tight-fitting wool tunic, somewhat soiled, displayed his broad shoulders.

He spoke in a pleasant, low-pitched voice. "Good morning, sir."

Michael returned the greeting. This must be Luke, allegedly Peter's cousin and Zosimas's victim. He was indeed handsome, certainly attractive to women and no doubt to some men.

But not to Zosimas.

"May I help you?"

Michael thought fast. Most men would send their wife or a servant to buy food. "I need some string."

Luke reached under the counter and brought up a basket. "Here's what we have—twine and string from heavy-duty to lightweight."

Michael looked through the contents, picked up a few balls and examined them, and eventually decided on a medium grade. "I'll take this."

Luke gave him a noncommittal nod. His thick hair fell into his eyes.

As Michael reached for his money, the voices in the back rose noticeably. Now he'd have to stall for time in order to listen.

One voice was male and raspy, with a slight Macedonian accent. "You shut up, stupid woman, and keep out of this!"

Michael feigned indifference and surveyed the barrels of fish and cheese, the crocks of wine and oil, and the baskets of dried beans and lentils behind the counter. Finally, he raised his eyes to the pottery on the shelves.

The conversation in the back room continued; another masculine voice—very deep—cut in, but Michael couldn't make out his words. Then he wondered: was the man even speaking proper Greek?

Finally, the poor, maligned woman spoke up. "I just don't want to—"

"Boian won't be staying," said the raspy voice. "He has to—"

Boian? A Slav, certainly. Most probably a Bulgar. Well!

"Er—I also need a new lamp," said Michael.

"I'll show you what we have." Luke tossed his hair back and took something down from the shelves. "Here." He placed a pottery lamp half the size of his hand on the counter.

"Thank you," said Michael, "but this isn't quite what I had in mind."

Luke grinned, revealing white, even teeth. "No decorations. Not the thing for a gentleman like you."

Michael suppressed a gasp. How much did they know about him? Maybe nothing. To a shopkeeper like Luke, perhaps everyone else was a gentleman. To Michael, on the other hand, Luke, regardless of his station in life, was a chunk of excrement.

Enough was enough. Michael took his changes, put it and the string in his belt pouch, and left. He'd continue his surveillance in a less direct way.

Once back outside, he took a good look at his surroundings. People came and went along the relatively wide Street of the Peacock. There were women shoppers with sacks and baskets, old-clothes vendor carrying their

155

goods over their arms or in handcarts, and linen-weavers who displayed their wares in the same manner. Candle shops, taverns and drinking booths—all well patronized, dominated the area.

For the time being, then, the neighborhood was safe. With so many witnesses on hand, Michael's unknown enemy would probably let him be. And in such a crowd, he would not be conspicuous.

He observed that the grocery, though flanked by a street on one side, had an alley on the other. The ground floor of the house across the alley also held a shop. But—what was more important—the entrance to the shopkeeper's private quarters would be in this same byway.

Just across the street from the grocery was a drinking booth. Michael headed straight for it and bought a cup of acidic watered wine. He joined the other customers who were lounging against the nearest building. They wore the dusty, dark-colored tunics of laborers. Michael must look no less disreputable, considering his passage through dirty alleyways, but had his disguise fooled Luke?

He tensed—he'd just have to be more careful—then settled down to wait. He sampled his wine and found it vile.

After a short while, he sensed more than saw a shifting shadow in the alley next to Peter's house. Then an austere, white-bearded man emerged onto the street, his eyes lowered. He wore a loose brown garment, a cloak of the same color, and a tall fur hat.

Had he come from Peter's house...or from the one next door. No, he must have come from the grocer's. His unusual headgear suggested the mysterious Boian. "Boian won't be staying," Peter had said.

The old man walked up the other side of the street, then turned into a candlemaker's shop. Minutes passed, but he didn't come out. Perhaps another quarter of an hour elapsed, and still he did not emerge.

Had he given Michael the slip? At least Michael would recognize the outlander if he saw him again.

For the present, Michael would do well to concentrate on Peter's store. No one entered by the front door, but after perhaps another quarter of an hour, something moved in the alley.

A smallish, stoop-shouldered woman, one edge of her cloak pulled over her head, came out of the byway. An empty sack trailed from her hand. Such a plain, defeated-looking woman could only be Peter's wife, the victim of his verbal abuse and stinginess.

Michael pretended to sip his caustic wine but watched her move up the street. Soon she disappeared into a candle shop—not the one Boian had entered—and emerged a moment later, dragging her bag along the dirty street.

As she shuffled up to a vegetable-seller's stall, Michael left his tin cup on the counter and set off in pursuit. He combed his hair back with his fingers, then took his signet ring out of his belt pouch and slipped it on his index finger.

What had she said? "I just don't want to..." If she disapproved of her husband's activities, she might be of some help.

When he was only fifteen feet behind her, he stopped short and waited until she'd dropped a couple of cabbages into her sack. He struck out again, narrowing the gap between them.

Unaware of his presence, she heaved the bag over her shoulder and entered a nearby bakery. He positioned himself near the door.

When she came out, her sack looked heavier. Well, what was wrong with buying bread? But though she kept her eyes on the cobblestones, Michael spotted a wine-colored bruise on her cheek. He clenched his teeth: so, the grocer beat her! He also noticed the pale skin of her face. It was set in countless creases.

How old was she? Michael didn't know Peter's age, let alone what he looked like, but surely her life with him had aged her prematurely.

He quickened his stride and caught up with her. "Good day, mother. May I carry your bag for you?" He spoke without dissembling; he'd been taught to respect his elders.

This elder jerked her head up like a frightened bird. Her mouth opened abruptly, like a beak. A puzzled look crossed her face. "Why yes, my son, thank you!"

"Where are you headed?" Michael asked although he knew quite well.

"That way." She pointed towards the grocery.

"I see." She had a native accent, unlike her husband.

Michael swung her sack over his left shoulder. "Let's be off," he said. "Ah, by the way, are you the wife of Peter the grocer?"

Her shoulders quivered. "Yes. Do you know him?"

"I don't know him personally, but I'm interested in his activities. I'm an agent of the Post." He showed her his ring.

Her pale eyes widened. "He's...in trouble?"

A strange reaction! Michael thought. Was she alarmed—or glad? "We don't know yet," he said. He would not give his name, or Bourtzes's, in case she told Peter. But somehow, he doubted she would.

"Promise not to tell anyone," Michael began.

"Oh, I won't."

"I have a simple question to ask. Was your husband at home Monday night?"

The lines around her mouth deepened, and she looked away. "No, he went out. Towards morning he came home drunk. He was with Luke."

"Luke?" What would she have to say about *him*?

"His young cousin, from the westlands."

"To which tavern did they go?"

The woman clasped her hands. "I don't know."

So! Peter and Luke had no alibi. Nevertheless, he would put her mind at rest. "Thank you, mother, and don't worry. I'm sure they've done nothing wrong," he said, though he thought just the opposite. "And remember—tell no one that we spoke."

Peter's wife gave him a weak smile. "I won't."

"Good." Either she was a consummate actress, or she bore her husband no great love. Michael rather doubted the former.

Now the high, red-roofed house loomed before them. He handed her the bag.

"Thank you," she said, and disappeared into the gloom between the buildings.

For safety, Michael joined a throng of shopkeepers and tradesmen who had come out on their noon break. Though he now relaxed his vigilance, his mind worked frantically.

Ever since his meeting with the Patriarch, he had suspected that both Peter and Luke were Bogomils, and everything he'd heard about them since then only confirmed his suspicions. Hadn't Bourtzes said that many merchants in Philippopolis belonged to the sect? How convenient! No one considered it odd if all manner of men went in and out of shops or travelled to sell their wares—men such as Boian.

But assuming that Peter and Luke were Bogomils, had they killed Bourtzes? So far, the only evidence against them was their lack of an alibi for Monday night. They were out carousing? Perhaps. But what if, instead, they'd killed Bourtzes? What if they knew that Bourtzes was pursuing the members of their sect? And what if they knew that Bourtzes had unearthed the plot against Father Zosimas? So they silenced him. It all made perfect sense.

Except for one thing: it was much too neat.

Chapter 20

I t was well past noon when Michael approached his back gate. He would change into some decent clothes, then ride out to the Studion.

But now he spied a two-horse carriage waiting in the street. Olympia's? His heart quickened.

No, this conveyance was grander than hers, with gold-painted trim. And he didn't recognize the eunuch in the driver's seat.

The silk curtains stirred. Moments later, a tall, beardless man in a blue garment stepped out—the Court physician. "Michael! Where were you?"

"Hunting down Bogomils and being shot at."

Again, the curtains rippled, and Michael heard a muffled feminine exclamation. So, she *was* here! He doubted, though, that she'd come only on his account. "Is there any news?" he asked.

"Bourtzes's cross is missing," said the doctor. "His widow noticed that it wasn't among the effects Lady Olympia returned to her. Nor was it buried with him."

"So!" said Michael. "We knew our list of his effects was missing something. Now we know what."

He fell silent as the carriage curtains parted, and Olympia Macrembolitissa, wrapped in a gray cloak, emerged.

He bowed low, attempting to conceal his appearance as much as possible. He must look like a sewer rat! "Good day, Lady."

"What have they done to you?" she cried.

"Nothing much." Emboldened, he looked up. So, she didn't find him disgusting. Then, like a soldier trying to impress his sweetheart, he recounted his trip to the grocer's.

She moved towards him. "Thank God you weren't hurt!"

Acropolites folded his hands across his paunch and smiled awkwardly.

Olympia exchanged glances with him, as if to say he wasn't intruding, then turned back to Michael. "What exactly did you find out?"

"Not much, but I'll wager that both Peter of Serrhes and his 'cousin' Luke are Bogomils. And they don't have an alibi for Monday night. Later I'll give you the details."

Acropolites nodded.

"Now I think we should go back to the murder scene and search for Bourtzes's cross," said Michael. "Just allow me to change my clothes." Alas, he doubted that he'd be able to see Zosimas today.

A short while later, they set off. Now on horseback, Michael led the carriage through the Forum of Constantine and along the Mese. There were people browsing in the arcade shops or exchanging gossip in the street. No doubt they took Michael for the servant of a great lord. Well, let them! He didn't mind as long as he could go about his business—and be near Olympia.

As they passed the tumbledown Wall of Constantine, the disc of the sun shone through an opaque, whitish sky, bathing the scattered, red-roofed houses and brownish slopes in its pale radiance. The distant orb presaged the coming of winter, but its beauty lifted Michael's heart. What lay beyond the veil of cloud? Light? Joy? On such a day, how could the Bogomils believe that an evil spirit had created the world?

Still, there was a blot on the sublime landscape: the skeletal branches of the beech grove.

"We're here." Michael called a halt and left his horse at the roadside, with the driver and carriage. As he led Acropolites and Olympia to the stand of trees, he told them more about Peter and Luke.

§

Somewhere downhill, dogs began to bark. "Stop yer yawping!" someone yelled. Michael smiled, recalling the farmers.

Eventually the dogs did stop.

Michael found the grove much as he remembered it. Underfoot, twigs snapped and decaying foliage groaned, while brownish leaves still clinging to their branches swayed in the wind. The depression at the center of the grove remained. His stomach pitched at the sight, and he tasted bile.

"Now all we have to do is find the cross." He felt a mounting sense of nausea, but, eager to set an example, he dropped to his knees, ignoring the dampness that seeped through his hose. Acropolites and Olympia too, despite the physician's protests, did the same.

They found nothing and fanned out towards the edges of the grove, turning up matted leaves, examining them in the cool light of sunbeams slanting in through the trees.

It was Olympia who saw a whitish light flash not four feet away from her. "Here!" She sprung towards the object

163

and picked it up. "Here!" she repeated, extending her cupped hand. Michael and the doctor stumbled towards her.

"Ah!" said Michael.

In Olympia's palm lay an eight-pointed silver cross on a chain. It was like Michael's own but larger.

"It's beautiful." He took it from her and wiped off the residue of dirt with his fingers.

"If his widow can identify it...," said Olympia.

"Um—yes." Michael's thoughts were elsewhere. He saw that the chain was broken.

He twisted the relatively large, rectangular links between his thumb and forefinger. "It must have been torn off, though it could have snapped accidentally. He couldn't have been strangled with it, could he?"

"No," said Acropolites. "It would have left distinctive marks."

Michael sighed. "I thought so." Minutes passed before he spoke again. "Still, it might be of use to us."

Acropolites inclined his head to one side. "How so?"

"Think: the cross was most probably yanked off Bourtzes's neck, thrown into the underbrush, and trampled upon. Which heretics despise the Cross, and instead of worship, give it every insult?"

Of course, they all knew the answer.

"The Bogomils," said Olympia. A fine line appeared between her eyebrows.

"And, as I've mentioned," said Michael, "I suspect that Father Zosimas's accusers are Bogomils."

"If so," she said, "they had a good reason to kill Bourtzes. And if the grocer and his cousin weren't home

Monday night—"

The doctor nodded. "It's quite reasonable."

Michael sighed. "However, there's a problem: what if the Bogomils did not kill Bourtzes, but the real murderer wants us to believe that he did? And so, he left the cross for us to find."

Olympia's shoulders slumped. "I thought you were going to say that."

"Oh well," said Acropolites. "My forte is medicine, not detection."

In any case, their work here was done. They climbed the hill towards the street, Michael and Olympia together with Acropolites trailing behind.

"Still, I don't think it was a waste of time to come here," said Michael, looking into Olympia's light-brown eyes. Being with you is enough, he thought.

"It was the only conscientious thing to do," she said. "Once we realized that Bourtzes's cross was missing, we had to find it."

Michael nodded. "Now we know that we're dealing with the Bogomils, or with a very clever foe in any case."

But now he stopped in his tracks. "Now that we're out here, there's something else we should investigate."

"Oh?" asked the doctor.

"There's an abandoned barn just to the west, somewhat closer to the street."

As they struck out across the slope, a grayish stone building, surmounted by blackish roof beams, loomed to their right. Scrub trees, matted underbrush, and dead weeds grew around it in patches. Otherwise, the dry earth was bare or covered with stones.

Just outside the ruin's gaping doorway, Olympia stumbled against a rock. Instinctively Michael grasped her elbow.

"Careful," he said, but he was the one who needed a warning. Even the feel of her sleeve, soft but well-worn, and warm to the touch, sent a tremor through him.

And what did she feel? She regarded him with luminous eyes.

But now they had no time for each other. They didn't need the doctor's promptings to enter the barn.

Inside, light poured in through the ruined roof, but the air was chill and musty.

"This place hasn't been used for livestock in a long time," said Michael, then noticed a pile of charred logs and ashes in a corner. "However, someone has been here recently."

"Vagrants, or the homeless poor?" the doctor wondered aloud. "It's a pity we don't have enough almshouses."

Michael nodded it. Yes, paupers could have sought shelter here, but he doubted it.

Olympia was near the far wall. "Look!" He approached and examined her find—a drying batch of horse dung.

"That can't have been here long," said Michael. "And paupers don't ride horses."

Acropolites laughed.

"No poor man sought shelter here," said Michael. "Perhaps Bourtzes was killed right here, and his body taken to the grove. Then the murderer—or more likely murders— seized his horse and took refuge in this place. They made a fire for light and searched his saddle bags. Then, not finding what they sought, they released his horse."

"No doubt you're right," the doctor said.

Michael took a deep breath and fell silent. Finally, he spoke again. "Indeed, this place can't be more than fifty feet from the street. So, it makes sense that Bourtzes was killed here, not in the grove. But we still have no better idea who killed him."

Later in the afternoon, they parted company at the ruins of the Wall of Constantine. Acropolites and Olympia returned to the Mangana in their carriage, but Michael, before heading home, made the short ride to the Inn of the Golden Fleece. He might as well try to see the Patzinaks again. Hopefully they had not yet left for their nightly carouse.

This time, when Michael pulled the bell chain, the proprietor himself, his key ring clanking, opened the carved double doors. He recognized Michael, and his florid face paled. "Ah—er—yes, Your Honor. What can I do for you?"

Though amused, Michael managed to keep a straight face. He wondered: was the fellow nervous simply because a government official had invaded his premises, or did he truly have something to hide? "I happened to be passing through the neighborhood and thought I'd check up on your lodgers, the Patzinaks. They're still with you?"

"Oh yes, Your Honor."

"If they're in now—"

"As a matter of fact, they just left." The proprietor motioned for Michael to come in.

They crossed the anteroom and paused in front of the

broad wooden staircase.

"So, they haven't changed their habits," Michael remarked.

The proprietor nodded eagerly. "Oh no, sir, they still go out late and come in towards morning."

"Do they still order a meal around noon?"

"Oh yes!"

Well, there it was! Michael could distinguish a regular pattern in their activities. And they had a plausible alibi for Monday night. No doubt they were still frequenting the Golden Gryphon tavern as well.

"You've noticed nothing out of the ordinary in their activities?" Michael continued.

"No."

Michael exhaled in frustration. "Thank you for your trouble," he said. Still, he thought it wouldn't hurt to stop by the tavern.

After leaving his horse at a guard post, he paused at the tavern door and looked westward, past the crumbling ridge of the old city wall. Scattered stands of trees, one of which was the beech grove, blotched the brownish slopes.

Still, the proximity of the Golden Gryphon to the putative murder scene hardly made the Patzinaks guilty. They could vouch for their whereabouts Monday night, and they were—ahem—busier than the other suspects, except perhaps for Saponas. And though Metiga was officially an ambassador, Michael doubted that he and Uzun had any serious business at court. They were here to enjoy the luxuries of civilization.

No matter; Michael would be thorough. He pushed open

the planked door and went in.

Two men glanced up from their chess game but returned to it at once. A raucous party of perfumed, oily-haired young fops at another table paid them no heed at all. There were no other customers.

But the proprietor, who was washing cups, recognized Michael at once. His facial muscles twitching, he put down his dishrag and hurried over. "Sir—er...ah—Your Excellency..."

"Good evening." Michael ignored the fellow's nervousness. "I'm asking after the Patzinaks again. Have they been in recently?"

"Oh yes, they come in every night—late! Last night I had to put them to bed again."

Michael groaned inwardly. What else had he expected?

Chapter 21

Though Michael wished he could have stayed home to rest, he presented himself at the Great Palace for the Emperor's function. It was held in the domed residence known as the Carian Pavilion, which boasted a vast reception room with walls of reddish Carian marble. Two or three dozen officials had come to eat, drink and exchange greetings with their Sovereign and Autocrator.

Among them, he recognized Saponas; his broad back was unmistakable. Where had he been this morning? Shooting arrows from a rooftop?

Of course, Michael did not expect him to own up.

Now he looked around the hall, nodding in satisfaction as he glimpsed Blachernites's white hair in the milling crowd. Michael would speak with him later, but first he must pay his respects to the Emperor.

As Michael crossed the room to His Majesty's seat, he saw that certain women, namely the Emperor's blond mistress, the Augusta, and her dark-haired attendants had been invited. There was no sign of the elderly Empress Zoe, who had been kind to Michael. But if Palace gossip deserved any credence, she had all but abandoned Court life and even her beloved perfume distillery for her icons.

Despite the purported informality of the occasion, the Emperor occupied a thronelike chair on a dais and received the prostrations and veneration of his guests. Several Varangian Guards stood behind him, while Constantine Psellus hovered nearby. A youthful, curly-headed eunuch, presided over a table laden with food and wine.

After prostrating himself, Michael hoped he could leave the Emperor's presence at once. For some reason his sensations were heightened. When the Emperor's chair creaked, it hurt Michael's teeth. Sweat trickled over his brow. He itched to wipe his face.

Indeed, the hall was much too hot. Several huge bronze braziers burned aromatic wood, and a working hypocaust warmed the floor.

But Michael was not about to be dismissed. "Stay!" The Emperor raised his large, gout-swollen fingers. "I have a favor to ask of you."

Michael bowed his head. "Your Majesty, I am at your service." Now he would learn why he had been invited; or was he being too cynical? Not long ago, he had saved the Emperor's life.

"I understand that you're on good terms with the Patriarch," said the Emperor.

Michael raised his eyes just enough to see that Monomachus had incline his blond head towards him. He heard the swish of silk garments as Psellus drew near—and shivered.

"One might say so." Michael would tell them no more than was necessary.

The Emperor did not speak at once but cleared his throat and shifted his scarlet-clad feet on his footstool. He waited for a eunuch to hand him a golden goblet set with rubies and sapphires, and drank deeply from it. When he was done, he passed it back to the eunuch and wiped his beard with a large red napkin.

Michael fumed inwardly. When would he get to the point?

"Furthermore, I understand that you've been called as a witness in a Church trial," Monomachus added in a low voice.

Michael startled but tried to keep his expression inscrutable. Well, of course they'd heard; it was no secret. "Yes, Your Majesty." But now what? Would the Emperor reproach him for not devoting his complete attention to Bourtzes's case?

"A ridiculous business, isn't it, defaming a saintly man like Zosimas."

Michael had not expected this. "Indeed!"

Psellus smoothed his mousy brown beard. "Yes, it's a farce."

"As Psellus may have told you," said the Emperor, "we think there's a way to stop the foul mouths of his accusers."

"Oh," said Michael. Yes, he'd heard about this scheme from the Patriarch. No, he did not approve.

But his lack of enthusiasm was hardly enough to discourage the First Secretary.

"These wretches can be threatened with exile—or worse," said Psellus, raising his bony forefinger like a blade. "If they don't withdraw their accusations by Monday, we can. Frankly speaking, I doubt that that good-for-nothing grocer and his cousin would enjoy being made eunuchs. Nor would those shifty monks, even though they've supposedly made themselves such for the kingdom of heaven's sake."

Michael snorted; no, they wouldn't like it. But he could hardly accept this solution.

Now he assumed a serious expression; he was, after all, speaking to the Emperor and his adviser. "Why don't you discuss this directly with the Patriarch," he asked, though he knew they already had.

"Oh, we did," said Psellus. "But we deemed it also advisable to talk things over with his staff, his friends, and with those who have standing in Zosimas's case."

Michael set his lips. So that was the strategy of the State: to put pressure on the Patriarch.

The Emperor leaned back and regarded Michael intently. "What do you think? Would the Patriarch agree?"

Playing for time, Michael took a deep breath. He disliked the tenor of this conversation—he was on edge anyway—but he could not afford to sound offensive. "Your Majesty," he began, "first of all, you know that the clergy abhor violence. And, in the second place, it's better to let the Church settle its own disputes. Don't you think so?"

Even as Michael spoke, Saponas's coarse voice rose above the buzz of polite conversation. "The monks of Mount Athos live a life of unequalled virtue. They don't allow women, or even female animals, in there." His audience, a bevy of eunuchs, giggled and tittered.

The Emperor inclined his head and listened. "Don't mind him. He's harmless."

"Under the circumstances, I hardly think so," said Michael, "not with an innocent man under suspicion." He tensed, and a red cloud hovered before his eyes. For a moment, Psellus's solution looked quite reasonable.

But no; such draconian action would do nothing to vindicate Zosimas. And the Church would never choose to be indebted to the Palace. Finally, Michael spoke again. "Your Majesty, I thank you for your concern." *But not for your solution.* "Still, it would be best to leave the matter to the Church. Let the trial take place and pray that Father Zosimas is proven innocent. Then no suspicion will remain in people's minds. On the other hand, if His Majesty were to intervene, it might reflect badly on—ah—the Court."

Psellus winced. "Certainly, one can do more than pray."

"Certainly," said Michael, "but coercion won't—"

The Emperor broke in. "You believe, then, that the truth will be revealed?"

"Yes," said Michael, though he knew that the truth often revealed itself in its own time, according to its own requirements.

The Emperor laughed graciously. "I can see that you're a man much like your master. I mean Zosimas."

"I wish I were, but I'm not."

"Well, God bless you. And good luck with Bourtzes's case. By the way, how's that progressing?"

Michael's heart sank, but he answered truthfully. "We have made...certain discoveries. We can say no more at this time."

"I'm sure you'll sort it out," said the Emperor. "You may go now."

Michael felt the tension ebb from his body. So, the Emperor was satisfied, at least for the present. Now, if only the Akoluthos would leave him in peace. "I thank you, Your Majesty."

After leaving the Imperial presence, Michael surveyed the hall again. The portly Saponas now stood at the long table at one end, heaping food on a gold plate. He was still at it when Michael came up behind him and tapped him on the shoulder.

Saponas looked behind him. "Ah, good evening, Taronites," he said, breathing wine fumes into Michael's face. "It's been so long since we've met—or a few days at least. I see you were talking to Psellus."

"Yes." So, the buffoon had noticed. Why did he care?

"Psellus always looks like someone shoved a poker up his arse, doesn't he?" Saponas's voice was none too low.

Michael did not reply, though he had to agree.

"What can I do for you? Won't you help yourself to some ants?" Saponas stepped aside, indicating a mountain of black caviar on a silver dish.

"Thank you." Michael surveyed the groaning table, covered with a purple-and-gold cloth. Beside the giant's portion of caviar lay dishes stacked with small, thin-cut rusks. Shucked raw oysters reposed on beds of ice obtained from deep within the Palace cisterns, or perhaps relayed from Mt. Olympus in Bithynia. Further down the table, mushrooms and dwarf olives swam in seasoned marinades.

Michael poured water and thick, purplish wine into a goblet. "I'm unaccustomed to such luxury," he said, intending no irony. He spread some caviar on a rusk and nibbled at it.

A eunuch, a young, sandy-haired fellow, ambled over to him. "Well, it's the best we can do, considering it's a fast day."

"So?" remarked Saponas.

Michael cast a sidelong glance at him. Was he drunk?

Certainly, his tongue had been loosened, though judging from everything Michael had ever seen or heard of the man, he was always jesting and spouting improprieties. "I was looking for you this morning," Michael said—never mind that it was not quite true.

Saponas slapped his thigh. "Too bad! I was out of the Palace then. I went home to check on my son."

And to shoot at me on the way to Peter's grocery? Michael struggled to maintain his composure. "Was he at home?"

"Oh yes. I also looked around the factory to make sure he wasn't botching things or violating the Eparch's regulations. I wouldn't want him to get his shriveled little butt flogged. Ha ha!"

Didn't this man take anything seriously? Michael made a mental note to visit the family soapworks as soon as possible.

"I found him managing quite well. Really, the boy's a regular drudge. He doesn't know how to enjoy life."

The eunuch looked up at Saponas. "Is life meant to be enjoyed, sir?"

Saponas roared "Of course!" and slapped Michael on the back. The wine in his goblet slashed dangerously close to the rim.

Now Saponas spoke in a hush. "In fact, I thought you should know. Someone here has been asking for you." He winked, then glanced across the room, towards the Augusta's ivory-inlaid couch. Her ladies-in-waiting surrounded it like dark blossoms.

The Augusta returned Saponas's look with a nod and

raised a beringed hand in greeting. One of her girls giggled.

"The Augusta is spoken for, of course," Saponas continued, "but the others are…available. I have it on good authority that any one of them would be pleased to meet you… And," he added in a whisper, "to sleep with the hero of the siege."

"The hero?" Michael pretended that he didn't understand, but he felt his neck grow hot.

Saponas must have noticed, for he poked Michael in the ribs; now his wine spilled on a Cathay carpet with a pattern of light blue flowers.

"Oops!" Saponas put in. "Why, you're the hero, of course."

Michael tried to think of a flippant retort, but Saponas forestalled him. "You can have whichever girl you want—or all of them, if you can take it."

The eunuch choked on his drink. Saponas, pretending not to understand the young man's discomfiture, pounded him on the back. "Come now, Eugene! Envy is never an admirable feeling. 'Thou shalt not covet thy neighbor's…doxy—or whatever.'"

Eugene's mouth formed a scandalized *O.*

Michael felt sorry for the eunuch and embarrassed for himself. "Ah—excuse me, I don't have time for this. There's something I must discuss with Psellus." He gulped what was left of his wine and turned to go.

Saponas snorted. "That pompous ass can wait. Allow me to introduce you to these lovely ladies." He grabbed Michael by the elbow and steered him towards the women. The hapless Eugene stayed behind.

Michael didn't protest. For the moment, he'd play along with Saponas and try to learn something useful. In any case, he knew a trap when he saw one. He was not so naïve as he'd been five years ago, when one of the Empress Zoe's maids had seduced him as part of a Palace conspiracy.

Michael bowed to the Augusta, who wore a narrow-cut dress of maroon silk. A gold belt with rubies, plus two gold chains, encircled her waist. Bracelets coiled around her sleeves like serpents, and the ornaments and gold wire in her upwound blonde plaits glittered in the light of the chandeliers. She was as lovely and as seductive as a heathen idol.

But now the idol shifted her position on the couch.

"Mi-chael, I haven't seen you since His Majesty's triumph, right after the siege."

The familiar form of address made him blush. "Ah—I've been busy." But though he must sound like a country yokel, he was no fool. He had asked her some very unpleasant questions during his first investigation, so why was she being friendly now? Had Saponas enlisted her in some scheme?

"Most August One..." Michael managed a polite smile. Then he became aware of the rustling of garments around him, and recalled why Saponas had brought him here.

The Augusta closed her dark, almond-shaped eyes. "My ladies-in-waiting wanted to meet you. They have heard so much about you."

It wasn't hard to guess from whom, Michael thought, as she introduced him with a sweep of her ring-laden hand.

The ladies—young girls, really—were dressed much like

their mistress, but with little jewelry. Also like her, they were from Alania, a land in the Caucasus, a client kingdom of the Empire. But their hair was black and hung loose and straight. Because it was natural, he found it more attractive than the Augusta's dyed tresses.

"Good evening," said Michael, and felt a flush creep up his cheeks.

He admired their almond eyes, their high, sculptured cheekbones, and the hint of small, firm breasts beneath their gowns. But they all looked the same, and he didn't know what to say to them.

"How long have you been here?" he asked one of the older girls. Still, she couldn't have been much over seventeen.

"Two year."

"Don't you ever get homesick?"

"Oh yes. I miss parents, but it's not nice place."

No, it was probably not a nice place.

Already restless, Michael cast a glance around the room, as he thought of another inane question.

Saponas, cup in hand, was chatting with two officials from the Fiscal Psellus, who had left the Emperor's company, glanced nervously at Michael, then joined Saponas, who was discussing drink. "The Russians guzzle slops called *kvas,* made from stale rye bread, while the Franks prefer a pig's swill called ale."

"What else can one expect from barbarians?" one of the Fiscal officials asked.

"Then there are the Tartars and the Patzinaks. They have their *koumis,* a brew made from fermented mare's milk. It tastes more like mare's piss. Ha ha!"

Psellus broke in. "Drinking that stuff is a perversion I'd thought beneath even you."

"I'd try anything once," said Saponas and exploded into a fit of laughter.

As all heads turned towards the group, Psellus managed a sanctimonious "Humpf!"

The awkward moment passed, and the guests began to mill about again. Michael excused himself from the women's company and headed back to the food table. As he refilled his cup and spooned some caviar onto a plate, he heard light footsteps behind him, then a dry, all-too-familiar voice. "The Emperor hardly needs a fool with him around."

Michael turned to face his superior, the Logothete of the Dromos. "Quite so. Er—good evening, Your Excellency." Oh, but he felt embarrassed! By now the Logothete must realize that Michael suspected him; indeed, the Varangians had questioned both him and his household.

"Good evening to you, Michael." Blachernites smiled urbanely, as if acknowledging Michael's discomfort.

Let him be innocent! Michael prayed. Indeed, why would the Logothete want Bourtzes dead? "Er—there was something I wanted to ask you."

"Would you care to meet me outside, where we can talk privately?"

"Fine. Where?" Michael narrowed his eyes. But the Logothete, even if he were a killer, would hardly lay hands on him right after he had been seen together.

"By the Baths of Theoctistus," said Blachernites and slipped away.

180

Michael wanted to speak to Psellus first but couldn't find him in the crowd. Saponas, he noticed, had joined the Emperor.

"Have you any new entertainments?" Monomachus asked.

"No, just some jokes. Have you heard the one about the eunuch and the abbess in the kitchen garden?"

"No! Tell me."

"Well..."

Some of the guests cocked their ears, avid for another of Saponas's filthy stories, but most people groaned and moved away. Nobody paid any attention to Michael, who slipped out of the room, feigning the impatience of one seeking the privy.

Though he was still warm from the heated hall and the wine he'd drunk, Michael threw on his cloak and hurried along a covered walkway leading to the marble-paved courtyard of the Sigma, the entrance to the Triconchus Hall. Here lanterns burned. Despite the chill, the fountain gushed light-colored wine that glittered like a shower of gems.

He left the courtyard through an arch and turned into a dark, narrow byway between the Baths of Theoctistus and the adjacent building. Soon he heard brisk, light footsteps on the marble flooring. His throat tightened. As he waited, his body tensed like a drawn bow.

It must be the Logothete, but what if it were his assailant? He had left his dagger at home because it was inappropriate to take a weapon to a social event.

The steps came very close, then stopped. "Taronites, is that you?" Whatever the Logothete's involvement in

Bourtzes's case, his brusque voice came like the blessing of dawn after darkness.

"Yes."

The Logothete's lithe form slipped into the passageway, his white hair and beard visible even in the gloom. "Good. Now, what did you want to ask me?"

"I was looking for you this morning..." Michael said, though it wasn't true.

"You must not have looked very far. I was in my office."

"Oh." That could easily be checked, but he doubted Blachernites was his assailant. "Er—I'm sorry, Your Excellency."

"What have you come up with?" There was the faintest hint of irony in his voice. "I haven't seen you for a while, so I don't know. Or am I being denied access to your information?"

"Not at all. And until today, I hadn't turned up anything conclusive."

"Oh?"

"This morning I went to Peter of Serrhes's grocery."

Blachernites eyed him quizzically.

"Peter is one of Father Zosimas's accusers. I didn't see him, but Luke, one of the alleged victims, was minding the store."

"Zosimas! What does that business have to do with Bourtzes's case?"

Michael bit his lip. What did Blachernites have against the monk? "Perhaps a great deal," he said, then related his narrow escape this morning. "And I just learned that Saponas was away from the Palace this morning."

"Why would he have shot at you? I still don't see—"

"Your Excellency, we now have Bourtzes's report. We know that the Bogomils are very active in Philippopolis."

The Logothete threw up his hands. "But I still don't see—"

"We also know that someone is interfering with the Patriarch's mail from the westlands, but he still gets enough of it to know that the people of Philippopolis want Zosimas to return there as their archbishop."

"And we also know from both Bourtzes and the Patriarch that the Bogomils of Philippopolis do not want Zosimas to return there as a bishop. So Bogomils here in the City are trying to prevent such a thing by slandering the future bishop. They could have also killed Bourtzes in order to seize his report."

"I see now."

"So, this Peter of Serrhes could be a Bogomil. So could his guests. Who knows—perhaps Saponas is also a Bogomil. In any case, neither of them has an alibi for Monday night."

The Logothete grimaced. "I admit—that makes sense. But what if your Zosimas is guilty?"

Michael glared at him.

"Sorry, but I'm entitled to my opinion."

"Yes." Michael felt that he could not completely trust the Logothete, so he decided not to tell him about Bourtzes's cross, an ambiguous discovery at best. For the present, let him think that Michael placed the blame firmly on Saponas.

"Well! You've been busy. Do you think we should arrest Saponas—now?"

My! He was eager! "I want more conclusive evidence first."

"All right." The Logothete furrowed his brow. "I'd better go now. You wait another few minutes, then leave." In an instant, he was gone.

Just as Michael stepped out of the passageway, he heard light footsteps in the Sigma. A shadow flitted towards him, and he returned to his hiding place.

The shadow halted a few feet away, and spoke in an accented, feminine voice. "Mi-chael, is that you?"

He replied in a hoarse whisper. "You!" It was Augusta's girl, the one he had spoken to. "What are you doing here?"

"I follow you and wait till your friend leave." Suddenly, she was in the passageway, pressing against him. He felt her hard little breasts against his chest.

He recoiled, but the instant passed, and fire consumed him. He slipped his arm around her and pressed her closer, caressing her cheek with his free hand. He lifted her face to his and sought her mouth. He had not been so close to a woman since—

An alarm began to clang in the distance—no, somewhere inside his head. No, not this time!

Shuddering, he flung himself away. The force of his flight flung her against the opposite wall of the passage. "Oh, sorry," he said. Wasn't he the gentleman?

The whites of her almond-shaped eyes widened in the darkness.

He seized her by the shoulders. "Who sent you?" he demanded. "Saponas?" Most likely.

"No one send me."

Michael tossed his hair back, and let her go. "Do you expect me to...believe that? Now...go!"

"But you like me."

He would have said something harsh, but he found breathing difficult. She seemed not to notice and retreated into the open. "Come here please. I show you something."

Wary now, he took a cautious step towards her, looking both ways before leaving the passageway.

She pointed downhill, towards a lighted window between two bare poplars. "I live down there, near my mistress."

"I see." Of course, she lived in one of the many women's suites in the Palace. At one time these quarters had been refuges for Court ladies and their retinues, where no males save eunuchs could enter. But nowadays they had become places where noblewomen and their attendants could receive their lovers.

"I go now," said the girl. "You come any time and ask for Susanna." She gave his hand a quick squeeze, then flitted away across a mosaic terrace and down some steps.

He watched her until she vanished. Something within him coiled tight.

Then, as he started back to the Sigma, he froze.

Footsteps! The sound of booted feet on marble.

Of course! She'd set him up for an assassin.

A chill sweat beaded his brow. Steady, he thought. The assailant had lost the advantage of surprise.

He slipped back into the passageway and looked out. A lanky, stoop-shouldered figure paused in the arched entrance to the Sigma. "Taronites," he called, "what the devil are you doing here?"

Psellus! Michael exhaled in relief. "Your Excellency! I was looking for you earlier."

Psellus approached. "Good! I see you got rid of the woman."

"Did you come to warn me about her? Who sent her?"

A shrug rippled Psellus's narrow shoulders. "I suppose I wanted to warn you. I saw her sneak out after you, and Blachernites left. I assumed she was up to no good, but I don't know who sent her."

"I can guess."

"Oh?"

"Saponas. Earlier he all but pushed me into her arms."

"Humpf! I saw... Now, what did the Logothete want?"

"A progress report, such as it was."

"Have you found anything to use against him?"

"No. I have no reason to suspect him of killing Bourtzes more than I suspect anyone else. I do know that he's no friend of Father Zosimas."

"Zosimas! I believe he's innocent as much as you do, but your job is to find Bourtzes's murderer." Psellus drew a breath, then fell silent for a moment. "And as you know, my Master and I are quite willing to help the monk."

"And as *you* know, the Church wants to settle the matter on its own terms. Moreover, the two cases may be connected, as I've said."

"What can I tell His Majesty?"

"The same thing I told him inside, which satisfied him. We've had some success."

Psellus snorted. "Success!"

"If anyone looks guilty, it's Saponas. This morning I was nearly hit by a sniper's bowshot, while he was away from the Palace."

"Really?"

"Syropoulos was also absent this morning, supposedly ill. And he wasn't here tonight. Was he invited?"

Psellus creased his brow. "He was. But wait—he *is* sick. You can't think—"

"He was at the meeting where Bourtzes's mission was discussed."

"But—the man's a snob, but he's an upright soul. What would he have to do with criminals, or Bogomil riffraff?"

"For the present, let's say only that not all his ancestors were so noble and pious."

"Oh." Psellus leaned toward Michael. "Exactly what t—"

But Michael no longer felt like talking. Of course, Syropoulos could be the hidden hand behind both Bourtzes's murder and the slander campaign against Zosimas, just as Saponas could.

Groaning inwardly, Michael raised his eyes to the vault of the night sky. There were almost as many possibilities as there were stars there.

But he knew one thing for certain: he would not go down the hill towards Susanna's light. And he would ask for an armed escort home. With such precautions, he might be able to keep his skin intact for another day.

Chapter 22

She came to him, a vision of white limned against the indigo darkness.

"Stay!" Michael kicked off the bedclothes, then lowered his feet to the floor.

She did stay—well across the room. Her diaphanous gown rippled in the breeze—what breeze? Through the garment he could see the outline of her body.

He drew a rasping breath. "Please, come here!" He moved towards her. His loins were aflame, nay, melting...

Almost imperceptibly, she nodded. He approached. Her hair shone through her scarf, but he could not see her face.

Who was she, anyway? Olympia? Susanna? Or a shade from the past—the Empress Zoe's maid, the one who'd seduced him... Ah, he had not forgotten.

"Now!" He reached. Her body glowed. No, it was transparent. Through it he could see the blackish square of the window. He clasped her arms, and his own hands showed through them.

Then she vanished.

He howled in frustration, then shuddered awake—a wake and alone. He lay supine on this bed, his body damp, the blankets tangled around his feet. A dim light crept in around the curtains.

He sat up, disentangling himself from the bedclothes, and kicked them away. "Damnation!" he muttered. He might as well get up and try to accomplish something.

He poured cool water into the copper basin on his bedside table, then wet a small towel and washed his face and body with it. Finally, after pulling on some clothes and saying his prayers, he tiptoed downstairs so as not to wake the servants. He didn't want to be fussed over and detained further. There was so much he should do today.

He must speak with Zosimas, who had concealed his plight. He would tell the monk a thing or two, though of course he would try to help him.

But first Michael stopped at the nearest bathhouse. He would cleanse his body, if not his soul.

So, after sweating out all but his life in the steam room, he dipped himself in the warm pool.

"A massage, sir?" an attendant asked him, when he came out.

"Not today, thank you." Michael flung a linen towel around his waist and walked on, eyes on the floor.

Then someone else hailed him: "Come have a drink with us." He looked up: some acquaintances, two other agents of the Post and a teacher of mathematics, beckoned to him from their poolside couches.

"I'm in a hurry," he replied.

He marched on to the cold room. Outside the windows, the trees in the garden danced and swayed; a stiff breeze had blown up. Nevertheless, he plunged into the great mosaic bordered basin, shuddering as the frigid water enveloped him, gasping as the wind gusted in through the open roof. He felt that his skin was being stripped away and found the feeling not unpleasant.

Later, once dressed and wrapped in his wool cloak, his cap pulled low on his brow, he felt pleasantly invigorated, but neither refreshed nor relaxed. Water, whether hot or cold, could not wash away what ailed him.

§

When Michael arrived at the Monastery of the Studion, church services were already over, and the monks had adjourned to the refectory. Along with the other guests, he was ushered into an adjoining dining room.

His companions were men of all ages and conditions: white-haired or hairless ancients, gawky striplings, paupers in rages, and gentlemen in heavy wool garments dyed in deep, strong colors. Many of them Michael knew by sight—he'd dined here before—though they'd hardly spoken. Silence was the rule during monastic meals.

After prayers, the guests took seats on the rough-hewn benches that flanked the several long tables. They bent over their plates of heavy earthenware and spooned cabbage stewed with salt fish into their mouths. From time to time they sipped pinkish watered wine from clay cups.

After a few minutes of this serious eating, Michael set down his spoon and broke a piece of the hunk of bread by his plate. Like the others, he strained to hear the reading in the refectory, the life of one of the saints of the day.

But another part of his mind followed its own course, observing and wondering.

Chapter 23

Andronicus Acropolites, the Court physician, had spent most of the morning in his office, writing. Lady Olympia and his assistants had the day off, and since he hadn't had any sick calls from the Palace, he was using the time to compose one of his periodic reports on the Emperor's health.

"Lately His Majesty's limbs and joints have been relatively free from inflammation," he wrote, "but there is no guarantee that evil humors will not flow into them again, deforming and incapacitating him utterly. Of course, if His Majesty would avoid women, wine, and rich fool, his chances of a relapse would be greatly diminished."

The doctor grimaced. The chances of *that* happening were minimal. Who ever followed his advice?

Acropolites marveled that gout could do so much damage. Had he missed the mark in his diagnosis? He dipped his pen into a silver inkpot and wrote out this last thought. Someone might find fault with his skill, but not with his courage.

What else could he say? He poised his pen and tried to compose his next sentence. Then he heard heavy steps behind him, in the doorway. Letting his pen drop, he sprang up.

The newcomer's low-pithed voice was familiar, its tone businesslike. "Good day, Your Excellency!"

Acropolites turned to face a shorter, stockier man: Lady Olympia's father, Basil Macrembolites. "I've come about my daughter," he said. His jaw, covered by a grizzled beard, jutted stubbornly. He advanced into the room with a firm stride, his silk garment swishing.

The doctor took a step backward, running his hand over his smooth chin. "About your daughter?" he asked, in a ringing contralto. "She's doing quite well. She's ready to be examined by the guild itself on our next feast day—you know, the unmercenary healers Sts. Cyrus and John, at the end of January."

Macrembolites nodded in evident satisfaction, but he did not smile. "That's not what I've come about."

The physician squared his shoulders. "Dear me! What then?" What indeed did this overbearing fellow want with him?

"Er—would you like to sit down?" the doctor asked, offering his guest a chair at the table by the windows. "Would you like something to drink?"

"No, thank you. This isn't a social call."

"As you wish." Acropolites sank back into his desk chair, where he felt more secure. Macrembolites pulled up his own seat.

"So—what can I do for you?" The physician shuddered inwardly. How much did the man know about Michael and Olympia's friendship?

"I'd like to know why your office has involved itself in an extremely sordid criminal investigation."

Acropolites bowed his head to conceal his surprise—and uneasiness. "You mean Bourtzes's murder." Alas, he'd tried to shield Olympia from certain facts of the case, but she'd guessed them on her own. Of course, she was an intelligent young woman. Intelligent and no doubt fearless.

"Now, since Bourtzes was an agent of the Post on a secret mission," he continued, "his death concerns the Imperial administration. So that's why our office was called in to determine the cause of death—and to search for anything on his person that might point to the killer."

"That's all very well, but—"

"Ahem—your daughter knows no more than she needs to." *And as much as she wishes to.*

Acropolites still didn't know if he'd vindicated Olympia—and himself. Her father was a judge and no fool. What if he knew about their expedition to the beech grove? And how much did he know about Michael?

The doctor folded his hands in his lap, out of the judge's sight, and twisted them.

Minutes passed before Macrembolites spoke again, a frown creasing his leathery brow. "I was not happy with her expedition to the house of Bourtzes's widow. She spent the night there... Oh, I know she was safe. She had our people— her eunuchs with her, but—"

"The widow needed a doctor's care."

"Why not you?"

"I thought that at such a difficult time, the widow would prefer to be attended by another woman. Lady Olympia returned Bourtzes's effects, and administered a sleeping potion. She spent the night there to make certain the lady was able to rest."

"Still, I'm afraid she's getting out of hand. She might do something to disgrace herself—and me."

"Oh. I see. I wouldn't think so."

Macrembolites tensed his squarish jaw, and studied his

soft leather shoes before he spoke again. "Well, I've always taught my daughters not to parade themselves in the public eye. And as for my sons, I've taught them to mind their own business and keep their hands to themselves. Ahem!"

The doctor startled. How much did the man know? He was surprisingly blunt, but why shouldn't he be? There were only men present—if one used the term loosely. "Now, that's certainly good advice, but your daughter's conduct is above reproach."

"Well, I can only hope that certain persons keep a close watch on the young men who visit their offices."

Acropolites made an effort to keep a straight face. So, the man knew something!

"I hear things. Has Taronites, the investigator, been haunting your office for the past few days?"

"Hardly that," said the doctor—which was the truth. "He's much too busy for that. But he does have good reason to consult with us."

Macrembolites held his peace.

"Please, I know you consider me...above suspicion," said the doctor, "otherwise you would never have entrusted your daughter to me. Indeed, I esteem the Lady Olympia as though she were my own daughter. I'm as zealous for her virtue as you are."

Acropolites watched the judge's face relax, then continued. "Now, if I did have a child of my own, either a boy or a girl, I'd raise him up in the same way I'm instructing your daughter: I'd teach him the art I know and love best."

The judge's voice was gruff. "I see you mean well.

Perhaps I'm the one who's been negligent. It's high time I arranged a marriage for her. In fact, I have a possibility."

"Oh?"

Macrembolites mentioned a name. "He's a judge in the civil courts."

Acropolites winced. "Sir, if I may express my humble opinion, it's always wise to proceed with caution where children are concerned."

The judge frowned again. "What do you know of that?"

"I'm hardly devoid of human feeling. And I was the son of a physician in a family of physicians. My father, who thought I showed more promise than my brothers, had me castrated. 'You're a genius,' he said, 'and someday you'll serve the Emperor. In *that* condition you can never ascend the throne, so he'll trust you.' I suppose he knew best. He was my father."

The judge's mouth worked. "How old were you then?"

Acropolites noticed the man's agitation. Good! he thought. I'll shock him into compassion for his own children. "I was around eight," he replied. I didn't understand what it was all about, but it was damned unpleasant."

Macrembolites actually shrank. "And later?"

"My mother died a few years later, then my father. As a youth, I was resentful for a while. But now I can see that I was spared much pain. No one had to marry me off."

The judge set his jaw again.

Yes, Acropolites thought, he understands.

Chapter 24

After the monastery meal, a bushy-bearded monk ushered Michael into a reception room furnished with a worn Peloponnesian carpet, a carved wooden settle, and matching chairs. The Abbot awaited him on one of these, leaning pensively on his staff. A humble man, he began to rise when he saw Michael. Forestalling him, Michael bowed to kiss his wrinkled, knotted hand.

"You wished to see me," said the Abbot, sinking back into his chair. "I presume it's about our dear Father Zosimas."

"Yes." Michael's hands hung limp at his sides.

"Please sit down."

Michael lowered himself onto the hard settle.

Smoothing his long, white beard, the Abbot regarded him approvingly. "His Holiness the Patriarch tells me that you'll testify in Father Zosimas's behalf—as will many others. Thank God for that."

"I'm hoping to prove him innocent."

"We appreciate that. I have no doubt of his innocence, though I was in the awkward position of submitting two of the complaints against him. I was appalled, but I didn't know what else to do. We have to follow canonical procedures."

Michael stiffened. "You're hardly to blame."

Noting Michael's discomfiture, the Abbot continued. "I didn't believe them then, and I don't believe them now. Father Zosimas is innocent."

Michael nodded.

"Despite the accusations, I too will testify in his defense."

"So the Patriarch said… And about your charges—the Novice Matthew and Father Jonas—I know they're lying, but I don't know why yet." He paused, feeling a spasm of inner pain; was he powerless to expose their falsehoods. "And the grocer and his worthless cousin are lying too!" Like boiling pitch, rage seethed inside him.

The Abbot groaned loudly. "*Kyrie eleison!* I know they're lying, but why?"

"I do have an idea about your people," said Michael. "Has either of them had a recent visit from a relative?"

The Abbot inclined his head in thought. "I don't think so. As you know, though we don't encourage such contacts, we don't forbid them. But I'm certain that no one has been to see either of them in a long time."

"What if someone from outside, not necessarily a relative, has made contact with them, and threatened them with something? What if they're lying under duress?"

"Under duress?" The Abbot shuddered and crossed himself.

"Please try to remember: have they had any visitors at all lately?"

After a brief pause, the Abbot replied. "I'm sure they've seen no one."

"One possibility remains," Michael concluded. "The monastery itself has many visitors—supposedly godly people who come to attend divine services. One of them could have brought in some odious message."

The Abbot blinked. "Woe is us if you're right."

"Today, in the guest refectory, I began to think: I recognized many of the men, but others I couldn't place. Though I'm certain that most of your guests are exactly what they seem, one of them could have been a wolf in the skin of a sheep."

"Alas!"

"In fact, I wonder if Father Zosimas has noticed anyone from his past life...someone with a grudge, or a family enemy."

The Abbot blinked again.

"Would you give him your blessing to accompany me to the Palace today? I'd like him to take a good look at certain officials...and to tell me if they've been here lately."

§

Michael found Zosimas in the cypress grove behind the scriptorium, huddled on an old stone bench. A too-large mantle, faded to an ugly dark green, was draped over his shoulders.

The poor monk! thought Michael. He was at loose ends, now, just waiting for the trial. And if he were found guilty, he would be expelled from the community.

"Father—"

Zosimas rose slowly and turned, leaning on his staff.

"Michael!" A look of mild surprise crossed his gentle, lined face, lightening his blue eyes.

"Why didn't you tell me?" Michael regarded him sternly. "I know I should have come sooner, but at least I've been spending time trying to clear you."

Zosimas flinched, and his veil fell back. Michael thought

that his hair and beard had grown whiter after the last few days.

The monk shrugged. "Why should I have told you? It would only have upset you."

"*Upset* me? Upset *me?*" Really, he thought, there were times when monks were utterly impractical. "Aren't *you* upset?"

"Yes, though I'm trying not to be."

"If you had told me, I could have assured you of my support, whatever that's worth. Certainly, you knew I'd find out eventually."

"And so you did. The Patriarch and the Abbot have informed me that you will testify on my behalf. Everyone has been very kind."

"Yes, but—" Michael drew closer to Zosimas, then threw his arms around him. Hot tears slid down Michael's cheeks.

Zosimas hugged him back; his chest heaved against Michael's.

Did the monk weep also? Perhaps this crisis prevented the sublime equanimity he strove for.

"I'm sorry, Father. I shouldn't have been so harsh." Michael straightened himself and wiped his eyes on the back of his hand. "But there is something we can do. Your accusers must be hiding some very guilty secrets."

Zosimas lowered himself to the bench again. "They must be."

"Can you think of any reason they wish to discredit you?" asked Michael, sitting down beside him. "I'm sure you've never offended them in any way."

Leaning on his staff again, Zosimas studied his sandals. "I tell you: I've never met this Peter of Serrhes and his cousin Luke."

"A year ago last summer, when you were on Mt. Athos, no shepherds came to sell their wares?"

"Some did, I'm sure, but I never had any contact with them. I mostly kept to myself."

Michael nodded. "I believe you. Now, what about the novice Matthew?"

"I know him by sight. He sometimes works in the same scriptorium but not with me. Indeed, I have no business talking to him. We're supposed to avoid the company of young novices—to prevent precisely the sort of thing that—"

"Do you know anything about him—his background?"

"He's from here in the City, isn't he?"

"Originally not. The Patriarch informs me that he's been living here with his aunt and uncle. They're weavers, but he was never apprenticed in that trade. Evidently, he's training to be a scribe... So, who are his parents, and what has become of them?"

Zosimas shrugged again. "I don't know."

"Now, what about Father Jonas?"

Zosimas took a deep breath. "I know him slightly."

"Now, I've learned that he's from a distinguished Senatorial family. But I can't understand what's turned him against you."

Zosimas looked him in the eye. "Then you have some idea about the others?"

"Perhaps."

The monk bowed his head. "About Father Jonas... You mustn't think that because we're monks we have no temptations."

Michael's whole body tensed. What was Zosimas about to confess?

Zosimas spoke in a pensive, dreamlike tone. "It happened back in the spring, on a warm, clear night. I was late leaving the church after Compline, and I cut around the back to go to my cell. Well, he was waiting for me behind the apse. He said he had to talk to me, so we started off in the direction of the scriptorium. I didn't think... I couldn't imagine... Then he...touched me."

Michael exhaled and said a silent prayer of thanks; yes, Zosimas was innocent! Still, his mind reeled from the shock. "And just last week he dared accuse you of committing the same sort of...mischief, and in the same place. Well! I gather you told no one."

Zosimas looked up. "He's a virtuous man."

Michael raised an eyebrow.

"Oh, I'm sure it was just a momentary weakness, that he's not given to that vice. I wanted to give him a chance to repent, without being exposed and shamed."

"Virtuous, is he?" Michael didn't know Jonas, and already he didn't much like him. "He acted with all the spite of a lover scorned. And really, do you think that if you had actually tried those things with him—and with the others— they would have shone you the same charity? You're turning the other cheek, but do you think for a moment that *they* would?"

"No, but that's hardly the point."

Michael tensed again. "Are you protecting Matthew as well?"

"I told you—I don't even know the boy."

"Ah—I thought his case was different. I suspect he acted under duress."

The monk's tone was noncommittal. "Do you think so?"

"Someone who wants to discredit you must have a hold over him. Someone had got to him here, with threats!"

"I don't know who would do such a thing."

"Have you noticed any strangers, any...unusual visitors to the monastery?"

"No."

"I have an idea why they are slandering you. I've been informed that you may be the next bishop of Philippopolis. The people want it, and the Patriarch is so disposed."

Zosimas smiled diffidently. "Oh, that's a great misfortune."

For the second time today, Michael regarded him sternly. "Come now! I hardly need to lecture you on the importance of your family. And who would be better than you. A sniveling careerist, or a secret Bogomil or Paulician?"

"Of course, if it came to that, I'd do my duty."

"I'm certain that the Bogomils are behind your difficulties. You would win over the people of Philippopolis and discredit the sectarians."

"Now, I was thinking they might be behind this slander, but it makes no sense. How can my accusers be Bogomils?"

"You know that the Bogomils keep their faith a secret. But I find something very odd about Peter the grocer and the company he keeps. And, as I said, I fear somebody is putting pressure on little Matthew."

"It's possible."

"Then please, come to the Palace with me now. I want to see if you recognize certain people, if they've been to the monastery recently."

The porter at the Brazen Gate admitted Michael and Father Zosimas without comment, but when they passed through the mosaic covered vestibule just inside, the Varangians stationed there greeted them with a puzzled gaze.

Michael was beyond caring. "Saponas, head of the Emperor's household, is our first suspect," he told the monk, as they emerged into a colonnaded courtyard flanked by high-windowed barracks. Their sloping red roofs added some small cheer to the sunless day.

"I think that Saponas is a Bogomil," said Michael, "as well as Peter and his so-called cousin. I also think that Saponas was orchestrating something last night, at the Emperor's reception."

Zosimas looked up. "You were there?"

Before replying, Michael glanced around. A servant swept leaves from the marble pavement; there was no one else. "I was invited," he said.

Still watching from the corner of his eye, he guided Zosimas off to the left, onto a tree-lined path. The broad golden dome of the Chrysotriclinium loomed ahead. "By the way, His Majesty inquired after you," he said.

"That was kind of him."

"Anyway, Saponas was there. He was—ah—making himself very much in evidence, and he practically pushed me into the arms of some women."

"Oh?" Zosimas stopped in his tracks.

"Yes, the Augusta's attendants—Alans, all of them. One of them followed me outside, and I'm certain that was Saponas's doing."

Zosimas looked away, and spoke in a strained voice. "I hope nothing happened. As you know, I can't hear confessions. I've been suspended."

Michael detected a note of bitterness in the monk's voice. He was trying to bear his troubles heroically but bending under the strain.

Michael placed a hand on his shoulder. "No, nothing happened. Still, you can advise me as a father, or even as a friend."

Zosimas faced him again; were there tears in his eyes? "I appreciate that. I'm not so strong that I can stand alone." He bowed his head. "What did you wish to tell me?"

Averting his gaze, Michael related everything that happened following his arrival at the Carian Pavilion the previous evening.

Zosimas nodded. "You say this...woman appeared to you in a dream? Indeed, I think it was only a dream."

"But very real."

"You were already agitated. I doubt you welcomed that...vision."

Michael raised his eyes to the bare branches and the leaden sky above. "Who can make sense of his innermost intentions and dispositions?"

"That's always difficult," said Zosimas, as they turned onto a marble-paved avenue. "Who can tell truth from falsehood, or virtue from vice. Sometimes they look the same—at least to mortal eyes."

"I should be better at distinguishing truth from lies than I am," Michael said. "After all, I'm an agent of the Post."

For a short while, they walked in silence; Michael was the first to break it. "But I want her still, the woman in the dream."

"You can't spend your life chasing phantoms, especially such—"

"I chase enough phantoms during my waking hours. Bourtzes's murderers, your hidden enemies…"

"That you can't help. But tell me, how is the Lady Olympia?"

"I saw her yesterday, ostensibly on official business. She always seems glad to see me, but—"

"As I've said, there are reasons a woman might not be eager to marry."

"It's much too soon to think of that. And perhaps I'm meant to be alone."

Zosimas wrapped his cloak around the lower part of his face, protecting himself from the rising wind. "Perhaps, but it's too soon for such a decision."

The wing of offices behind the Chrysotriclinium loomed ahead of them. Soft light shown from several of its arched windows.

"The Logothete of the Dromos is in today," said Michael. "We should call on him."

"I know him by sight already," said Zosimas. "He comes with the Emperor when His Majesty visits us on the Beheading of St. John the Baptist."

"Has he returned since, by himself?"

"No. He hasn't been in the church, anyway."

"Oh," said Michael, disappointed. "Then we'll find Saponas."

They rounded two more corners of the octagonal building, then paused before the embossed, gilded bronze portals the marked the entrance to the Emperor's private apartments.

"Is Saponas here?" Michael asked the pair of Varangians at the doors.

The elder, who recognized Michael, uttered a phlegmatic "Yes," but regarded Zosimas with narrowed hazel eyes. "Who's your companion?"

"Come now! He's a monk and quite safe."

"All right." The guard shifted his iron axe from one shoulder to the other and nodded them inside. They crossed the inner courtyard, stopping before the pointed cypresses that screened the kitchen door.

Michael spoke in a low tone. "If I'm right, Saponas is here. The kitchen is a favorite place of his."

"Now, Michael…"

"We'll just sneak in and take a look. So much the better if he doesn't see us."

Zosimas did not reply but simply followed Michael along the wall.

Today the door was closed against the raw weather, but past it was an unglazed window whose shutters hung open. Michael peered in cautiously.

The kitchen was much as he remembered it, with assorted pots, pans, spoons, and knives hanging from the low ceiling. And, just as before, the kitchen smelled of smoke and onions. The man who worked there was gutting mackerel and throwing the offal into a bucket. His wife fussed over a large earthenware baking dish.

Saponas, Michael saw, was amusing himself. He sampled crocks of wine sloshing some of each into goblets made of silver or colored glass. "Not bad," he'd say, smacking his lips.

Michael withdrew from the window and motioned for Zosimas to take his place. The monk did so.

Michael heard Saponas snigger, then break into raucous laughter.

After a few moments, Zosimas turned away, looking pale and slightly sick. "Let's go," he said.

Michael assumed that Saponas had been pinching or pawing the woman.

Finally, Zosimas spoke. "I've never seen the man before, not at the monastery or anywhere else."

Michael's spirits sank; another of his theories proved fruitless.

"An interesting man," said Zosimas. "'This kind cometh not forth, but by prayer and fasting.'"

"I doubt that Saponas has ever done much of either."

"Well, you never know."

Somewhat disheartened, Michael led Zosimas back out of the Palace, to a bench at one edge of the Augusteum, in the shadows of the Patriarchate, where they had a good view of the Brazen Gates. No one leaving the Palace would escape their notice.

All they needed to do was avoid attracting attention to

themselves—a simple matter. People wandered through the square, browsing in the perfume-seller's stalls, or queuing up at a street vendor's brazier.

Indeed, thought Michael, what could be more natural than a monk and a layman conversing outside the Patriarchate? They weren't the only ones; close by, a group of monks and Palace officials were discussing the errors of the Latin Church.

"The Spirit cannot proceed from both the Father and the Son," said one monk. "That doctrine destroys the unity of the Godhead."

"I don't quite follow you," said a courtier in a fur-lined cloak, "but it *is* nonsense. It's nowhere mentioned in the Scriptures."

Zosimas had been following their conversation. "We haven't heard the end of this yet. I understand that the Patriarch is quite concerned."

"And so he should be. But there's another insane doctrine that matters to us more, at least at the moment: how can anyone believe that the devil created the world?"

The monk leaned toward him. "Is it that hard to understand, when the devil's activity is so much in evidence? And if one does not believe that the devil created the world, the origin of evil is more difficult to explain."

Michael wanted to ask another question when the clock in the Augusteum sounded its low-pitched *bong*.

"Wait—" He drew a deep breath and counted out nine rings. The gold-embossed Brazen Gates swung open, and a handful of men in heavy, gold-trimmed cloaks emerged, seeking their servants.

"We'll see if you recognize anyone," said Michael.

"So far I see no one."

Michael slumped his shoulders. "We'll wait a little longer."

And surely enough, the shining gates opened once more, sending forth a tall, well-proportioned man with a dark beard. A large gold brooch held his sable-lined cloak in place.

"Aha! Speaking of the devil—"

"Don't," said Zosimas. But he watched the newcomer, who now surveyed the Augusteum with a haughty, impatient gaze.

"That's Leo Syropoulos, the *Kanikleios*. Have you ever seen him?"

"No. Or, I may have seen him at the monastery with the Emperor, but that was a long time ago."

Michael exhaled in exasperation. Still, they continued to watch Syropoulos until the latter spotted two men—servants, no doubt—and a pair of black horses, and waved them toward him.

"You know, his family has a very interesting history. His ancestors were Paulicians, a fact that he tries to conceal."

"Can you blame him?"

Michael was about to speak, then drew in his breath. One of the servants, a slim, beardless youth in a fur-lined cloak, handed Syropoulos a conical sable hat. The boy then mounted one of the horses. The other servant, gray-headed and dressed in dark-colored wool, held the reins of his master's horse until the latter swung into the saddle and took the reins. Then, with the servant walking several paces ahead, Syropoulos and the youth rode out of the square.

"He's an arrogant man, to be sure," said Zosimas, "but that doesn't make him a Bogomil or a murderer."

"But what about that boy? Who's he?"

"I've seen none of them at the monastery."

"Syropoulos could have sent someone else."

Several times more, the Brazen Gates flashed open and shut. Among those leaving, Michael saw the Logothete of the Dromos, but not the last man he sought.

The Gates had closed for the day: the clatter of bolts and bars echoed across the Augusteum.

Finally, Michael spoke. "Do you know someone called Gregory Tripsychos?"

Father Zosimas raised his head. "No. Should I?"

"Things would be much simpler if you did."

Chapter 25

Michael had seen Father Zosimas safely back to the monastery, but now, as the indigo darkness descended around him, Michael reached the drinking booth across from Peter of Serrhes's grocery. Though the latter establishment was closed, the former was still busy. Men lounged on the cobbled street, gulping wine from tin cups and eating the salted chickpeas that filled a bowl on the counter.

Keeping his eyes on the house across the street, he sipped—or pretended to sip--the wine stall's vinegarish swill. He observed narrow bands of light around the shuttered window and beneath the front door. Peter's strange family was probably cleaning up.

Michael laughed inwardly at himself. What did he expect them to be doing—preaching Bogomil servants on the corner, or sitting on the roof, sniping at passers-by?

He'd just have to wait for their next move. He was certain that Peter was up to no good...and that there was some disagreement between the grocer and his wife.

The sky turned darker, and a wind began to blow. Michael pulled his wool cap low over his head and huddled into his cloak. Perhaps a quarter of an hour passed. Then the metal gong in a nearby church began to sound for Vespers, causing a flurry of activity along the street. Lights were doused; doors slammed. People shuffled into the street, towards the clanging.

The zone of light around Peter's window vanished.

Well, now what?

Moments later, two people emerged from the alley next to the grocery. One wore a woman's baggy cloak and gown, with a plain kerchief. She kept her shoulders bowed, her eyes on the cobblestones. In her Michael recognized Peter's downtrodden wife.

The other figure was a man, though not the mysterious, striking Boian. Of medium height and stocky build, he wore a short cloak over a shapeless tunic. His face was bearded.

Michael nodded in satisfaction. This must be the notorious Peter of Serrhes.

Peter walked ahead of the woman. Around them more lighted windows went dark, doors opened and shut, and people spilled outside.

But the patrons of the drinking booth didn't budge an inch. Could Michael leave without attracting attention? He'd have to try: he left his cup on one end of the counter, and, with an air of feigned nonchalance, ambled off, pulling his cap even lower over his forehead.

He quickened his pace, then stopped short, allowing several people ahead of him. He fell in about twelve feet behind the grocer and his wife. He could distinguish them well enough; Peter, he noticed had fair hair, a broad Slavic face, and a prominent nose. Aside from his stocky build, that's how Michael would recognize him.

As he followed them, he passed the candle-maker's shop where Boian had disappeared yesterday morning and recognized the store that Peter's wife had entered. Further up the street were other groceries, their shuttered windows dark. But some other doors still hung open, belching forth the stench of sour wine and salt fish, as well as coarse laughter.

Another fifty feet, and the pair would be at the church. Michael hung back, but kept them in sight. Would Peter actually go in?

He did, and his wife followed. Michael joined the worshippers pouring in through the double doors. He paused in the narthex only long enough to take off his cap, then peered into the glowing darkness of the nave. Men stood elbow to elbow, but he could not find Peter among them.

Michael slipped inside and stayed in the shadows of the back. Beneath the curves of the dome and its supporting squinches, the soft light of the lamps and candles illuminated the frescos on the wall and the bowed heads of the men. He did not see Peter or his wife; presumably the latter had gone up to the gallery with the other women.

The service had already started. The reader was concluding the opening psalm, which praised the goodness of God's creation. How would a Bogomil react to that? Michael wondered. Of course, he would keep his feelings to himself.

People shifted their positions, then fell silent as the deacon took his place before the Royal Doors, at the center of the iconostasis, and began the litany. Michael moved forward, positioning himself behind a column, and looked around. He could see better now. In the lamplight, one of the bareheaded but cloaked figures looked familiar. Was it the grocer?

When the litany was finished, the men shuffled their feet. Some coughed. One tiptoed to the rear of the nave, but he was a frail, bent fellow, not Peter.

Then another man elbowed his way through the crowd, stopping only in the front ranks of the congregation. Michael recognized his sandy hair and stocky frame.

So the grocer was playing the pious churchgoer. Didn't he ever make a false step?

Chapter 26

Sunday noon found Michael in the atrium of Hagia Sophia, waiting for the Emperor's retinue to leave the church after services. He huddled into his cloak as the wind blew a few stray leaves across the marble pavement.

Last night, when he'd arrived home, he'd been surprised to find a message from Acropolites asking him to please come to his office around the ninth hour. At the time Michael dared hope the physician might have discovered something important.

At that time, he decided to attend services at Hagia Sophia on the following morning; it was just up the hill from the Mangana and Acropolites's office, and just across the square from the Great Palace. He just might have a chance to speak with a certain elusive courtier.

That morning Michael had looked through the church's dusky expanses towards the *metatorion,* the gold-latticed enclosure occupied by the Emperor. The high officials of the Court surrounded it—among them the Logothete of the Dromos and Leo Syropoulos.

Curious! Syropoulos had been at the Great Palace yesterday and was here today. He appeared completely recovered from whatever had ailed him on Friday.

But now, as Michael stood in the atrium, the central outer doors of the narthex swung open. The noisy throng around him fell silent and parted.

Borne on fragrant clouds of incense and the sonorous chant of many voices, the Imperial procession came forth like a comet crossing the sky. The courtiers in their gold trimmed robes were first; then, surrounded by Varangian guards in scarlet, Monomachus walked as though on swollen feet. His leonine head was bowed under his heavy crown, and his shoulders slumped beneath the gleaming *pallium* that hung from his neck. The Master of the Universe looked none too well.

One the procession had passed, the people broke rank, bustling about in search of friends or family, resuming their conversations. But Michael of course did not join them. "Excuse me," he said, elbowing his way through the crowd. He followed the Emperor's entourage into the Augusteum, then hung back until it had disappeared into the Palace. He sat on a stone bench near the Brazen Gates and hoped that Syropoulos wouldn't take long inside.

About a quarter of an hour later, the gates opened, and half a dozen courtiers came out. They had doffed their robes of office and now wore heavy wool cloaks, some lined and trimmed with fur, over long wool garment, some bordered with gold embroidery. After exchanging good-byes, they set off in different directions, no doubt in search of their servants. Only one of them, the tall, imposing Syropoulos, remained by the portals. Today he wore a different cloak pin, set with a large cabochon ruby. Again, he scanned the square impatiently.

Michael jumped up. He must reach the man before he mounted his horse. If they were both on foot, Michael might have an advantage.

But the *Kanikleios* walked past Michael's bench.

"Your Excellency!" Michael called.

Syropoulos looked back. "Ah—it's you. What do you want?"

"I'm glad to see you're feeling better. I heard you were ill on Friday."

Syropoulos's black eyes smoldered. "What business is it of yours? Yes, I was, as a matter of fact."

"It must not have been anything serious. I know, because I saw you here yesterday."

"I had a stomach ailment."

"You were home sick all day Friday?"

"Yes! May I ask why—"

Subtlety would serve no purpose with this man, Michael thought. Bluntness, on the other hand, might shatter his arrogant façade. "You hadn't gone to visit your friend, Peter the grocer?"

"Who? What are you talking about?"

"Peter of Serrhes. He has a shop in the Street of the Peacock."

"Never heard of him!"

Michael heaped one provocation upon another. "And I suppose you've never heard of Father Zosimas either."

The *Kanikleios* scowled. "What do I have to do with some damned sodomite monk?"

Michael dug his fingernails into his palms, stifling an impulse to punch Syropoulos in the nose. "How dare you call him that? Especially you, with your little friend!"

"You scum!" Syropoulos made a fist, but Michael raised his own in defense. He studied his face; did the man's olive skin blanch? "Perhaps you're the one who started those rumors."

"What nonsense!"

Then a youth's voice called out, "Your Excellency!"

It's the pretty boy, Michael thought. I must hurry. "What if spreading evil gossip helps your family interests?" Michael continued.

There was a glimmer of uncertainty in the courtier's eyes. "What are you talking about?"

"I know why your forefathers tried to pass themselves off as Syrians."

Syropoulos paled, then turned an apoplectic shade of red. "What do you mean?"

The few people who lingered in the square now turned their heads. Then—

"Master—" The dark, smooth-cheeked boy grasped Syropoulos's wrist. The youth's cloak swirled about him, exuding the musky scent of patchouli. "Trouble him no more," he told Michael.

But Michael did not allow Syropoulos to escape him. "Many of my own ancestors were Armenian," he said, "and I don't hide the fact. None of them, however, were Paulicians."

Syropoulos blinked but held his peace.

Michael lowered his fists and nodded, satisfied. So the courtier's ancestors embarrassed him! "I know all about Gregory of Argaoun."

"But he came over to us." Syropoulos's swarthy, angular features were composed once more, his mask of politeness in place.

Michael raised an eyebrow. "Then you have nothing to hide after all."

218

"No. Now, if you'll stop this harassment—" Guiding the youth by his elbow, he turned his back to Michael.

"I won't keep you from your...amusements," Michael called after them, "but I have one more question: where were you last Monday night?"

Syropoulos looked over his shoulder. "Home!" Then his obsidian eyes widened in understanding, "So you're the one who sent the Varangians to question me."

"Yes. What do you know about Bourtzes's death?"

Syropoulos set his lips so that his dense whiskers nearly covered them. His shabby middle-aged servant approached, leading two horses by the reins. "Your Excellency—"

"Enough!" Syropoulos and the youth mounted, wheeled their beasts around, and kicked them hard. The hapless pedestrian servant hurried to keep up with them.

They behaved as though Michael did not exist.

§

Around the ninth hour, Michael presented himself at the Court Physician's office in the Mangana Palace. The door had been left ajar, and Acropolites was sitting at his desk, reviewing documents. The windows had been shuttered, and a rack of lamps lighted the room.

Michael knocked, and the doctor rose. "Michael, come in." He gestured towards the table. "Have a seat."

Michael pulled up a chair. "Your Excellency, do you have any news?"

"Nothing much to do with the case, but I did want to tell you this. On Friday, after we parted, I sent one of my assistants out to St. John's hospital, to see if Tripsychos went there for treatment Monday night."

"Since you don't seem particularly elated, I presume he did go."

"Yes—during the second watch of the night. They cleaned his wound and changed his dressing, just as he said."

"Still, he had some leeway...even though, with his injury, he couldn't have—"

"But you've decided that Bourtzes's killer had help."

"It's probable."

The doctor went over to a cabinet and returned with a pitcher of wine and two cups. "You're not ruling out Tripsychos?"

"I'm not ruling out anyone yet."

Acropolites poured a cup of wine for Michael and passed it to him, then sat and poured one for himself. "Er—I did have a note from Lady Olympia yesterday. She took the cross we found to Bourtzes's widow, who confirmed it was his."

"Good. That doesn't help us much, but at least it's not a setback," said Michael, then looked at his cup. "Is there any water?"

"Er—you're going to need this. About Lady Olympia—"

Michael startled. "Is she well? What about her?"

The physician sighed and examined his cup. "Yesterday morning...her father came to see me..."

Michael felt the news like a kick in the stomach; what would he hear next?

"The esteemed judge thought that our office was taking an undue interest in a sordid criminal case. I assured him that though the Bourtzes affair was our business, it wasn't really his daughter's concern."

Michael took a hefty swallow of wine. "That wasn't quite truthful."

"What else could I say? I was trying to protect you both."

Now it was Michael who bowed his head. "Thank you."

"He also inquired about Lady Olympia's association with you. Of course, I told him that it was well-chaperoned—by me—and purely professional."

"It's not much more than that."

The physician sipped his wine. "I may have pacified him for the time being, though he plans to make a match for her."

Michael drew in his breath.

"He mentioned the name of a judge in the civil courts. But fear not—I hear all sorts of gossip, and what I don't hear, I can find out. Many people's private lives don't bear close scrutiny. I can discover what dirt they're hiding, and pass on the news. Lady Olympia's father is certainly hard-headed, but he's an honest man. He doesn't hold with evil doings."

"Thank you for letting me know. But I'm helpless. For her family, I simply don't exist. And it's probably utterly presumptuous of me to even think of—"

The physician arose and placed a hand on Michael's shoulder. "Oh, I think she likes you well enough, but there are reasons a young woman might not wish to marry."

Michael laughed. "The last person who told me that was a monk."

Acropolites resumed his seat. "Is that so?" he said with

a chuckle.

Michael nodded.

"Well, surely you've noticed what marriage is like among people of our background. The husband is busy with his position, his property, his colleagues. When it comes to offspring, he's around for a few moments, at the beginning, and then foists them on their mother, on nurses and tutors, and servants—"

"Are you telling a dirty joke?" asked Michael, pouring himself more wine.

"It's not a joke. It's the truth."

"My father spent a great deal of time with me."

"Your father was an exceptional man, may God rest his soul," said the doctor. "And you too are exceptional."

Michael sighed. "Hardly that."

"Take heart," said Acropolites, setting down his cup. "I'll do what I can to help both you and the lady."

Michael rose from his seat. "Thank you for warning me and for the news you brought me. I feel as though I've reached a dead end. I haven't found Bourtzes's killer, and I have yet to expose Father Zosimas's slanderers. Yet his trial begins tomorrow, and I must defend him."

The doctor followed him to the door. "May God guide us all."

Chapter 27

Monday morning, when the pale sun hung low in the east, Michael set off for the Patriarchate, arriving in the atrium of Hagia Sophia well in advance of the third hour, the time set for Father Zosimas's trial. Already a great number of men and women had gathered there. Many of them wore the fine, fur-lined cloaks of the wealthy, but most wore the coarse wool wraps of the common folk.

Michael understood that they were here on account of the trial, but how many of them were for Zosimas, and how many against him?

Though some people stood off to one side, chanting hymns, a large throng exchanged noisy abuse and curses.

"That dirty bastard monk..." said one fellow, adding unnecessary details.

"Shut up! Yer a sodomite yerself," an old woman flung back. "Yer all lying."

Setting his teeth, Michael stepped into the fray, searching for someone friendly, or at least rational. He spotted an older man in plain but clean clothing, a man who was neither swearing nor shouting, and approached him. "Good morning, sir. What brings you here?"

The fellow straightened himself. "We heard that they're going to try Father Zosimas, but we know he's innocent. His Holiness should know."

"I'll tell him. Indeed, the Patriarch also believes he is blameless."

"But *those people* have come too."

Yes, thought Michael, evil tongues always spread their filth. "Fear not," he said. "Father Zosimas will be cleared." Alas, if he were only so certain! "But you and your friends should pray for him."

"We will, but..." The man's eyes widened. "You know the Patriarch?"

"Er—yes. And we both believe that the monk is innocent."

"Good."

Michael scanned the crowd, then turned back to his ally. "Father Zosimas isn't here yet, is he?"

"No, Your Honor."

Michael dreaded what would happen when the poor monk did appear. He was glad to have pleasant company now.

But even this comfort was soon denied him. A strong feminine voice—not Olympia's—called out. "Michael, is that you?"

Now who—

He turned. A dark, petite woman, with a little boy at her skirts, was waving to him. Though she looked familiar, Michael could not quite place her.

"Excuse me," he said to his erstwhile companion, and made his way towards her. "Yes, Lady..."

"You haven't changed a bit," she said, "but I can see you don't remember me."

She was quite young, though her clothes and headgear largely concealed her physical attributes, except for a lock of dark hair that fell over her brow. When he drew closer, he knew her by her soft black eyes.

"Barbara!" Yes, he knew her! A little over five years ago, she had been the Empress Zoe's maid, and she had seduced him. A mistress of the then Emperor, Nicknamed Michael the Caulker, she had acted as his pawn, as part of a plot to discredit Michael's father. And once Michael had learned of her circumstances, he forgave her. No, that wasn't quite the truth: he had always blamed himself.

"How are you?" he asked. He cast a discreet glance at the small boy.

"I'm well, thank you. And this is my son Symeon."

Michael recalled having heard that she was married; in fact, immediately after the overthrow of Michael the Caulker, the Empress Zoe had taken Barbara under her wing, giving her a dowry and making a match for her with a Palace pastry cook.

Michael ruffled Symeon's hair. "Hello, there!" The boy gave him a crooked smile, then hid his face in his mother's skirts.

Michael felt a blush creep up his neck. Assuming a formal manner, he addressed Barbara again. "What brings you here?"

Her eyes brimmed with tears. "We didn't want to see an innocent man condemned?"

Michael startled. "You knew him?"

"My husband met him once or twice. But he couldn't come this morning. He had to work. But we both believe that Father Zosimas is innocent."

"I *know* he is. I was called as a witness for him."

Barbara wrapped her head-covering tighter around her face. "I'd heard."

"I'll do my best for him, though I'm afraid that's not much."

She reached out and clasped his hand. "You always did your best."

He blushed. Did I? he wondered.

And what did she want with him now? Was she trying to seduce him anew?

He put away the thought. How uncharitable could he be? "I hope, at least, I tried my best."

She opened her mouth to speak, but something forestalled her. A cultivated, very familiar voice, called out to him from afar.

He looked over his shoulder, in the direction from which the voice had come. Olympia had just come into the atrium—and waved. With her was Acropolites, his blue cloak thrown jauntily over his shoulders.

Michael felt a twinge of uneasiness; had she seen him with Barbara? How much explaining would he have to do?

He waved to Olympia, then turned back to Barbara. "I must speak with you later," he said.

"I won't be troubling you any more, sir," said Barbara.

"You're not!"

Insist though he might, she lowered her eyes and put an end to their conversation. Some people nearby began to cheer, but not for them. Others threw out jeers, catcalls, and rude noises.

Like everyone else, Michael looked towards the columns of the atrium. A group had just entered; he could make out Father Zosimas's compact form, as well as the gray-bearded figure of the Abbot. "Excuse me," he said, "I have to—"

He crossed the atrium and joined the group of monks. Zosimas, he thought, did not look well. The finely-lined skin of his face had a pale, unhealthy cast. And though his expression was cheerful enough, the deep creases around his mouth betrayed an underlying strain.

"Michael!" asked Zosimas. "Why are all these people here?"

"Because most of them care about you! They know you're innocent."

"I see." The monk's blue eyes were moist, and he quickly looked away.

They made their way from the atrium to entrance to the Patriarchate, but a barrage of taunts welcomed them. "Bugger! Pervert!"

Zosimas drew a rasping breath.

"Pay them no heed," said Michael. Instead, it was he who looked back. More people were joining the rabble. No doubt Father Jonas, the novice Matthew, and Peter of Serrhes, were among them.

No! thought Michael. They mustn't get away with this.

"Look!" One of the monks with Zosimas motioned into the distance. There, with the measured gait of women, another dark-clad procession approached.

Zosimas squinted against the strong light, and a smile spread over his face. "It's my sister. She wrote to me and said she'd testify."

Michael was glad for him. Zosimas's sister was now the abbess of a convent on the west side of the City. But years ago, when she had been the wife of an officer in the Excubitors, Zosimas, then a young student, had lived in her house.

As the two parties converged, the abbess—Mother Anastasia—exchanged the kiss of peace with her brother, Michael noted the family resemblance: blue eyes, a sturdy but compact build, and strands of fair hair growing white.

"I hope they'll let me testify," she said.

"Why shouldn't they?" said the Abbott of the Studion.

Father Zosimas replied. "Because she's my—"

He never finished the sentence. Others had been watching, and someone behind Michael made an obscene remark.

The nuns gasped in outrage, but one of them—an ageless crone, gave as good as she got. "Shut your filthy mouth!"

Michael felt a surge of anger and spun around. *Now they'd done it.*

He saw the culprit—a scrawny fellow in a dark-colored cloak—and slammed his fist into the man's face. Michael ignored the man's grunt of pain and seized him by his garment, then pushed him away, feeling the rough wool tear. "You lying son of a bitch! Take that back!"

"Ooooh!" exclaimed the crowd.

"Michael!" said Zosimas.

Michael's blood pounded in his head. *He* was not about to take anything back. He waited, hands on his hips, until the slanderer pulled himself to his feet, until he'd wiped the thick blood from his nose with the edge of his cloak.

Michael, calmer now, took a better look at him. He was thirty-five at the most, with an undistinguished, patchy beard.

"That's Father Zosimas's sister," he said. "Are you going to accuse him of incest in addition to everything else? You'll apologize, or I'll—"

Cringing, the fellow looked at Michael, then at Zosimas and the Abbess. He bowed hastily, then backed away, blood still trickling over his lips.

Michael pulled a handkerchief from his belt pouch and threw it at him. "Here! Now get out of my sight!"

The troublemaker immediately lost himself among his own people, who cheered and slapped him on the back.

The monks cleared their throats and shuffled their feet.

Eyes lowered, Michael turned back to them. "I'm sorry for my outburst," he said, bowing eloquently to them and the nuns. "But I couldn't just stand there and let him—"

"Serves him right," said the ancient nun.

"Who was he, anyway?" Zosimas inquired.

"I've never seen him before," said Michael. "Obviously he's a pawn of your enemies."

Mother Anastasia pursed her lips.

Once more, Michael scanned the crowd. A few people were staring at them, but by most were either chanting hymns or talking among themselves.

"I think we might as well go in," he said.

"Like Daniel, into the lion's den," Zosimas added.

As they approached the bronze double doors of the Patriarchate, the throng surged around them. "Back," warned the doorkeepers. "Only those with a standing in this case are allowed."

Just before Michael went in, he spotted Acropolites and Olympia standing near a group of noisy onlookers. Both were pale, neither spoke, and Olympia clenched her hands.

Chapter 28

The spiritual court took place in a chapel in the Patriarchate. Michael came in at the rear of Zosimas's party and saw the six judges—all bishops, including the Patriarch, seated at a table in front of the icons. They faced the nave, where a number of benches and chairs had been set up.

Zosimas and the monks with him occupied a bench near the tables, and Michael found a chair behind them. He looked around the church to see who had come. Mother Anastasia and her nuns settled on a bench behind him, and now others were arriving.

First came a group of several monks, whispering among themselves. The Patriarch nodded towards them, knitting his heavy brows. Michael guessed that Father Jonas and the novice Matthew were among them.

Michael tried to compose his thoughts. He wanted to believe that Father Zosimas had nothing to fear—first of all, because he was innocent. Indeed, both the Patriarch and his abbot believed so. In addition, he believed that the dark-clad bishops now facing them were impartial; they came from dioceses near the City and knew neither Zosimas nor his accusers. Indeed, if Zosimas thought any of the judges prejudiced against him, he could challenge that judge's competence to hear his case.

People were still filing in. But where were Peter of Serrhes and his notorious cousin? What if they'd changed their mind and had withdrawn their accusation?

But no: two men in plain but clean wool tunics and hose

strode in and bowed graciously to all present. Michael recognized the stocky, large-nosed Peter of Serrhes as the man he had seen in church Saturday night and the younger man, supposedly Luke, as the one in the grocery. This latter, in an effort to look respectable, had combed back his thick, chestnut-colored hair.

A buzz of conversation filled the chapel, and the Patriarch stood up and gave the people a stern look. Then he bade everyone stand for the opening prayers. Afterwards, the judges turned back to the people again and motioned for them to sit down. The Patriarch lowered himself gradually into his chair, as though in pain, and began shuffling the many documents on the table. "Priestmonk Zosimas of the Studion?"

The monk rose. "Here am I."

"Have you been duly informed of the charges against you, and the identity of those who made them?"

"I have, and I've read copies of their statements."

"How do you wish to answer these charges?"

"As God is my witness, I'm innocent. You've read my own statement. I brought a copy, in case..." He extracted several parchment sheets from the depths of his robes and waved them.

"Very well, but first we must consider the accusations brought against you." The Patriarch winced. "The first is lodged by Peter of Serrhes, a grocer with a shop in the Street of the Peacock. Peter?"

The grocer stood up, managed a shallow bow, and sat down again.

"The complaint is lodged on behalf of his cousin Luke,"

said the Patriarch, and read as much of the ill-composed statement as he could. "Er—most of this is written in language unsuitable for an ecclesiastical court."

The people rustled their garments.

"Now, Luke…" prompted the Patriarch. "You can speak for yourself. You're not mute."

Luke now stood.

"Is this statement true?" asked the Patriarch.

"Yes, Your Holiness."

Zosimas regarded the youth calmly. Michael thought that Luke shrank, or at least hunched his shoulders. "I've never seen you before," he declared.

Peter blurted: "Of course you'd say that!"

"Can anyone corroborate this story?" one of the bishops asked. "Have there been any other reports of Father Zosimas's…unsuitable behavior on Mount Athos?"

"No," said the Patriarch.

"I was on Mount Athos," said Zosimas, "but I never met this youth, if he was ever there."

Now the Abbot broke in. "I received a letter from a monk there who described him in glowing terms."

In the back of the room, someone laughed nastily.

Michael looked back, but failed to discover the culprit. He turned back to the Patriarch. "Please, Your Holiness, people might think that Peter of Serrhes is a good, man, but he's a whitewashed sepulcher, full of rot and dead men's bones."

"Please explain yourself."

"He beats his wife," said Michael.

"What of it?" someone demanded.

"How do you know?" asked the Patriarch.

Michael tensed. He didn't want to reveal his encounter with the grocer's wife. "The neighbors see her bruises and hear him cursing at her."

The bishops shuffled their feet unevenly. "The neighbors didn't bring this to our attention," one of them said.

"See?" Peter demanded.

"So, I just brought it to your attention," said Michael.

"Well," said the Patriarch. "Whether or not the neighbors consider this behavior reprehensible, we do."

Again, the people began to talk among themselves in angry, indignant tones, and once again, the Patriarch silence with an upraised hand. "Of course, it's possible that we've overlooked something," he said, "but does anyone know any reason why Peter of Serrhes should not testify in this court?"

A murmur rippled through the church, then subsided.

"I know a very good reason," said Michael. "His cousin is not a child and can speak for himself. And there's more—"

"That will do for now. You'll have a chance to speak." He exchanged a quick glance with Michael, then picked up another leaf of parchment. "Now, let's consider our next document..."

"The next complaint against Father Zosimas has been submitted by the Novice Matthew, of the Monastery of the Studion..." He read part of the statement and summarized the rest. "So, he maintains that Father Zosimas approached him in the scriptorium, at the beginning of July, when just the two of them were there."

Matthew, a slender young man, stood up. "That is correct."

Michael scrutinized him. Though he was heavily swathed in dark robes, his clear dark eyes and curly beard, still thin in some places, were visible. He was a handsome youth, just as Luke was.

But the novice appeared to be ill. Though the chapel was cool, his face was slick with sweat.

Now Zosimas spoke up. "Young man, this is simply not true. I know you by sight, to be sure. You worked in the scriptorium, but we never worked together, and you were never left alone with me."

"Yes, I was," said Matthew, "several times. Each of us worked on his own project. I never thought he'd—"

"Not so!" said Zosimas. "Perhaps you worked alone there, just as I did. But we never worked there at the same time."

Michael had definite reservations about this youth. Something was not as it should be. "Please," he began, "may I ask him some questions?" His eyes met the novice's dark, liquid ones. "You're not a native of Constantinople, are you?"

Matthew gulped down a breath, then spoke. "No, but I've lived here for eight years. Before I entered the monastery, I was with my aunt and uncle."

"Their names," prompted one of the judges, the Bishop of Cyzicus.

"Artemios and Martha of Didymoticus, residing in the Street of the Weavers. They work in wool."

Michael arched an eyebrow. "So you're from the

westlands. How did you come to live with your aunt and uncle? Are you an orphan?"

Matthew looked down at his sandals and squeezed his eyes shut. "No, but my parents are poor peasants who made great sacrifices to send me here, to school."

"So your parents are still living. Have you any brothers or sisters?"

At this point the Bishop of Cyzicus broke in. "What has this to do with the witness's competence?"

"Perhaps a great deal," said Michael.

"You may continue," said the Patriarch.

"My siblings died in infancy," replied Matthew, "but my parents still live."

"And they're poor peasants?" asked Michael.

"Well, yes. They have a small farm near the foothills of the Balkan Mountains."

Just as Michael suspected! "That's not the most secure part of the Empire to be living in these days, is it? It was recently in the clutches of a rebel would-be emperor. And as if that weren't enough, it's a seed-bed of heretics, and it has been ravaged by the Patzinaks. Also, like the rest of the Empire, it's terrorized by private tax-collectors who threaten the poor."

"This has nothing to do with the matter at hand," put in someone next to Matthew.

"Doesn't it?" retorted Michael.

The Patriarch nodded.

"Your Holiness," said Matthew's companion, "this man is hardly above reproach. Before court opened, this fellow swore at a man and hit him."

People began to whisper. "Is this true?" the Bishop of Cyzicus demanded.

The Abbot of the Studion rapped his staff on the floor. "Taronites, the gentleman in question, was extremely provoked. The man he struck had made an indecent remark about the defendant and his sister, a nun of holy reputation. Such a ruffian would not have listened to reason."

"Are you condoning such methods of solving disputes?" A thin, sallow-complexioned monk spoke up.

"That's Father Jonas, the third accuser," someone told Michael.

"No, I don't approve of such methods," said the Abbot. "But in this case they're understandable."

Somebody guffawed. "If that's the kind of defenders Zosimas has—"

"Quiet!" put in someone else. "What's going on? Hey—he's fainted!"

"Who?"

"The Novice Matthew."

Matthew's place on the bench was indeed empty. Several people huddled around, it muttering among themselves.

Michael nodded, certain of one thing. Matthew's accusation was a lie.

"The court is closed," said the Patriarch. "We will reconvene tomorrow at the third hour."

Chapter 29

After parting company with Father Zosimas, Michael could not decide to go to his office or home to rest. He did feel exhausted, completely poured out, after two of the accusers had spewed out their filth. Still, the situation was not hopeless. He was certain that when he did have the chance to speak, he could discredit Peter and Luke. And Matthew had acted strangely, then swooned. Michael was certain that his testimony was a lie.

Now, Father Jonas and his testimony must still be dealt with. Michael did not like the look of the man; he had the sanctimonious air of a pseudo-ascetic.

Zosimas simply must be proven innocent, Michael thought, as he stepped out of the atrium of Hagia Sophia. If the charges were dropped simply because his accusers couldn't prove them, they still would have won. Then, even if he were elected Bishop of Philippopolis, a cloud of doubt would overshadow him. And the Bogomils of the Empire, in their underhanded, sniggering way, would point fingers at him as typical of the thorough corruption of the Church.

Yes, he must be proven innocent. Then he would put the heretics to shame—not by his words, but by his example. He would—

"How was it?" A pleasant, medium-pitched woman's voice broke in. *Olympia's.*

Michael turned. Olympia, her gray cloak pulled tight around her head, stood near one of the columns.

He bowed deeply. "You're alone?" Where were her

eunuchs? And where was Acropolites?

"I saw you here this morning."

He startled; could she say no more? But he answered her eagerly. "Yes, and I saw you!"

"Oh? Yes, you did." She fixed her light-brown eyes on him. Her question was closed, impenetrable. "The doctor and I went back to the office, but he let me come back to see what was going on."

He recoiled as though stung. *Was that all?*

"I wish I had something more conclusive to report," he said. "But so far, the case against Father Zosimas is not absolutely damning."

"But it can't be—if he's innocent."

"Exactly! I know he is, and I gather the judges think so as well, though of course they're trying to be unbiased. But so far, we can't absolutely prove that the plaintiffs are lying. And the witnesses for him have still to testify."

"Well! I certainly hope that you can vindicate him."

Again, Michael felt a sting of pain. "Are you dismissing me?"

She lowered her gaze. He adjusted his own to meet it and saw her squint to contain her tears. "Olympia, what?"—

"Look, I know this is none of my concern…"

How formal! He changed his tone to match hers. "Lady Olympia, I'd like to think that whatever it is *is* my concern, and yours also."

"Before the trial, I saw you talking to a woman. Is she your mistress?"

He choked back a cry of dismay. "My *what?* No!"

"No?"

He did not wish to dredge up that part of his past, but he wouldn't hide it either. "I won't dishonor you by lying. There was something between us long ago. But I haven't seen her since. She has her life, and I have mine."

Olympia turned away. Her words rang clearly as a bell, and echoed in his mind. "I thought I saw something in you. But you're no different from other men, who take their pleasure where they may, and—"

"It's not as you think! I blame myself entirely, and I haven't forgotten. Please understand: it was a trap, part of the case they made against my father."

"How can I believe that?"

"I have not lied...though I'm hardly as guiltless as Zosimas, or my father."

"I can't—" A sound between a cough and a sob muffled her words. She hiked up her skirts and ran towards Hagia Eirene, in the general direction of the Mangana Palace.

"Can't you understand?" Michael called after her. "Can't you forgive me?" Only when she was out of sight did he stir. He found walking difficult, as if his feet were shackled, but he forced himself to push ahead.

Have I truly lost her? he wondered, as he headed up the Mese. No, it could not be!

He turned down a side street with a few respectable taverns and chose the first one he saw.

A waiter was wiping the shiny wooden tables as Michael came in. Several groups of Court officials had arrived before him and were waiting to be seated. "Come join us," one or two of them said, but he pretended not to hear.

He slouched over to the counter and sat down. Except

for a man utterly absorbed in his drinking, he was alone.

The proprietor approached Michael. "Would you like to order a meal?"

"Barley porridge, beans, stewed octopus, cabbage with salt fish—"

Michael's stomach twisted. "Er—no thank you. Just bring me a small jar of red."

"Water on the side?"

"No."

He paid, and immediately applied himself to the wine, which he drank from a plain pewter cup. He sampled the dishes of salted chick peas and lupines on the counter.

Woe! He had not apprehended Bourtzes's murderer; he had not cleared Father Zosimas. And now he had surely lost Olympia.

His mind was divided in two. One part wished to continue the fight, but the other wanted only to forget.

He poured himself another cup of wine and downed it, but it did nothing to ease his tension. Like the rope securing the throwing arm of a catapult, he was being wound tighter and tighter.

He took some more chick peas, swallowed them forcibly, then wiped his hands on his handkerchief. Food disgusted him; he'd limit himself to drinking.

Just when his taught facial muscles began to feel numb, the stench of sweat and horses enveloped him. What in hell's name was *that?*

He turned. A man with long black hair, and a shaggy beard stood over him. He wore an unusual coat of light-green silk, with a split skirt.

Michael rubbed his eyes. If he were any drunker, he'd think he was seeing demons. As it was, the fellow looked familiar.

He clapped Michael on the shoulder. "You here?" He smiled broadly, showing his flawless white teeth.

"Ah, of course!" By now Michael had placed him. "Honorable Metiga! Fancy meeting you here."

"I was thirsty."

"So was I."

Metiga stepped up to the counter and ordered his own crock of wine. Without bothering to retrieve his change, he took the jar and two cups. "I be seeing you, hey?" he said, as he headed toward a dark corner.

Chapter 30

Impelled by a dire need to use the privy, Michael woke in the dark, with an aching head. Where was he?

He rolled over. The lumpy feather mattress felt familiar. Of course. It was his own.

Once he was completely awake, unpleasant memories whirled through his mind. He'd been drunk, and though he'd been capable of making his way home, he'd vomited up all but his soul in an alley. He had taken a foolish risk; what if his mysterious pursuer had caught up with him in that state?

And, what was worse, the outcome of Zosimas's trial appeared uncertain. And Michael had most probably lost Olympia's affection…for telling her the truth about himself.

And, and, and…

And finally, he had neglected Bourtzes's case.

But had he? He sat up with a start. Perhaps not. Perhaps he'd been allowing ideas to ripen in his mind.

He recalled seeing Metiga in the tavern, with a wine crock and two cups. At the time he was too drunk to react to the Patzinak's presence, but now he wondered…

He stumbled out of bed, made his way to the window, and pushed the curtains aside. The sky was growing lighter.

He'd make up for his lapse. He'd discover what the Patzinak had been doing in the City center, around noon—a very early hour by his standards.

But Michael's day was already full. As soon as he dressed, he planned to visit Saponas's son, in the soapmakers' district. He hoped that afterwards he'd have time to check in at the Great Palace before the Church court convened. He hoped he could testify today.

§

A zone of orange flamed across the dark eastern sky, warming the chill, acrid air of the Street of the Soapmakers. A militiaman directed him to Saponas's house, which was three stories high and boasted a blank stucco façade. It was the sort of residence that the wealthiest citizens would have found adequate, if the rear wing hadn't contained a soap factory and if the neighborhood weren't so full of stench.

Michael pulled on the bell chain. Within minutes, the double doors swung open and a servant appeared. "Yes, sir?"

Striding into the tile-floored vestibule, Michael flashed his signet ring. "I'm an agent of the Post, and I'd like to speak to the young master."

The servant bowed low and donned an obsequious smile. "He's back in the factory, Your Honor."

Michael followed him down one or two long corridors, past a row of windows opening onto an interior courtyard, into a vast-high-ceilinged chamber. Despite the lamps and candles placed throughout, the air was thick and hazy. Heavy smoke and steam ascended from vats and cauldrons, then vanished through open windows and vents in the roof.

Michael breathed cautiously. The tang of lye, partly masked by olive oil and heavy perfumes, was not the best thing for his disordered stomach.

Once he'd grown used to the odors, he ventured inside and addressed a worker stirring jasmine essence into a vat filled with an indescribable mess. "I'm looking for your

244

employer."

"Over there." The man indicated a gigantic copper pot with a fire underneath.

A slender, sandy-haired young man stood near the urn, his back to Michael, and examined its contents. "It's cooking all right now," he said to a laborer in attendance.

"Saponas?" Michael inquired.

The youth spun around, wiping his hands on a plain brown tunic. "Yes, I'm Mark Saponas, and who might you—" He looked Michael in the eye but didn't shrink. "Listen, if you're from the Eparch's office, you'll find nothing out of order here."

"I'm not from the Mayor. I'm from the Post." Michael displayed his signet ring again.

Young Saponas's gray eyes widened. Though a light-colored beard covered most of his face, he looked quite boyish, uncertain and unjaded. And there was something else about him.

"But we've already been searched," he said. "You must have sent the Varangians."

"I did, but I saw no harm in asking you a few questions myself."

Mark frowned—and looked five years older. "Then I presume this is about my father. About the Bourtzes murder."

"Yes. As you know, we're concerned that your father has no alibi for last Monday night. And we understand that he wasn't here. Now, please, don't think that you're under suspicion, but where were you at the time?"

"I was here—or in my living quarters. My wife and

servants can vouch for me. In fact, the Varangians already asked me that."

"I was just checking. I'm more interested in your father. Are you on good terms with him?"

Mark shrugged. "I think so, but I don't see him much these days. He devotes all his time to the Palace, and I run the business now."

"Is he happy with that arrangement?"

Mark scratched his beard in thought.

At last Michael realized what was extraordinary about this young man: he had pockmarks on his forehead and on his broad cheeks, which his beard didn't quite cover. Michael now recalled that Ingvar had mentioned the scars.

"I think Father prefers to be where he is."

"I see," said Michael. Ingvar had also remarked that the younger Saponas was as likeable as the elder was vulgar and unpleasant. Michael quite agreed, and an ineffable feeling of compassion welled up in him.

"Does your father come to visit you often?"

"He was here last Friday, for the first time in ten days. He didn't stay long."

Michael nodded; this was important. "At what time of day did he come?"

"Early in the morning. He said that he just came to see me—and to make certain I wasn't botching things. Then he was off again."

This was exactly what Saponas had told Michael at the Emperor's reception. Since the former soapmaker did not stay long at home, he could have had enough time to position himself on a roof near Peter's grocer, which was no more than a few minutes' walk from here. And here he could have obtained a bow and arrows. He could hardly be seen leaving the Palace with such equipment—and without a good excuse.

Mark creased his scarred brow. "Has he...done something else?"

"He may have. But there's no point in worrying about it yet."

"*Kyrie eleison!*" Mark crossed himself. "My father's a criminal!"

Michael placed a hand on the soapmaker's shoulder. "Not necessarily. I'm just trying to form a better idea of his manner of life."

"Just what do you wish to know?"

Michael feared that what he was about to ask would further undermine the young man's confidence in him. "Ah—does your father have a mistress?"

Mark flushed. "I... I don't know. He'd never tell me, anyway. But I've often wondered...ever since my mother died, and especially ever since he went to work in the Palace, he talks...like he can have any woman he wants."

So! Perhaps Saponas *had* been with a woman the night Bourtzes was killed. Then again, Saponas's amorous exploits might be no more than talk.

"Does he often go out at night?" Michael continued.

"He didn't when he lived here. I have no way of knowing what he does at the Palace."

"Hm." Michael thought there was something else he needed to ask. "Your mother—she's been dead for how long?"

"My mother, God rest her soul, died ten years ago. She—she had the smallpox." Mark's gray eyes brimmed with tears.

"A dreadful scourge," said Michael.

"My brothers and sisters, they... Only I..."

Michael seized him by the shoulders, then embraced him. "You alone survived. And your father."

"He didn't get it," Mark sobbed. "He often wondered why."

Michael released him. "Some people simply don't." He shook his head in wonder. He could understand, though, how one might explain the phenomenon: Saponas was so offensive that not even the smallpox would come near him.

§

Michael reached the Augusteum well before the third hour, when courtiers, Palace employees, and the idle curious were just beginning to converge on the square. He entered the Palace through a guarded postern and, soon afterwards, reached the plain, whitewashed office of the Akolouthos of the Varangian Guard. Michael didn't relish speaking with him, but he trusted him more than the Logothete of the Dromos.

"Has the situation changed since Friday night?" Michael asked.

The Akolouthos set down his pen and ran his fingers through his short blond hair. "Not so far as we know." He raised his cool gray eyes to Michael. "What have *you* learned?"

Michael shuddered inwardly. How could he conceal his lack of progress? "I've ruled out no possible suspects, but

Saponas looks guiltier than ever. However, I find it curious that—"

"You found what curious?"

"Yesterday noon I happened to meet Metiga, the Patzinak ambassador, in a tavern near here. I rather doubt he comes this way often, at least so early in the day. Had he been at Court?"

The Akoluthos made a face. "Yes, he was with his brother. He petitioned His Majesty to take further action against his people's enemies, the Patzinaks of Tirakh Khan."

Michael suppressed a sigh. "I knew it was something like that."

Chapter 31

This morning Father Zosimas's trial convened in the same chapel as yesterday, and the testimony of the plaintiffs or accusers continued. "We will now consider the testimony of Father Jonas, a monk of the Studion for fifteen years, a man of good repute who has been deemed worthy of the priesthood."

Many members of the assembly shuffled their feet, sighed or drew breaths, but uttered not a word. Among them was the Abbot of the Studion.

Michael, who today sat beside Zosimas, studied Alypios. He knew that the monk was guilty of much, but in any case, he wouldn't have cared for the fellow's looks. Gaunt, with angular features pinched in what resembled pain, he appeared to be a sanctimonious type—a false ascetic, as Michael had thought yesterday.

But he decided to save his missile for the right moment, when the target came well within range.

The room grew silent. The Patriarch huffed, and waved a document in front of him. Then he resumed speaking in a weary voice: "Father Jonas, according to his statement, was passing by the scriptorium late one night, and heard questionable noises from an open window. He entered the building and went into the room, where he allegedly saw Father Zosimas *in flagrante delicto* with an...ahem...unidentified individual. Father Jonas states that the alleged culprits escaped through the aforementioned window before they could be apprehended."

The Patriarch interrupted himself, fixing his dark eyes

on the accuser. "So, this is how it happened?"

"Yes." Father Jonas raised his gaze to the judges. His skin had a grayish, grimy cast. "That's precisely how…" He pulled at his beard. "I just can't…"

"You find it painful to speak of," one of the bishops remarked. "Now, that's understandable. And this youth over here looks positively ill."

Michael glared at the Novice Matthew, who appeared to be examining his sandals. Even so, he could see that the youth's face was pale.

Had he deceived the bishop? Michael didn't think he could be such a fool.

But perhaps Matthew *was* frightened sick—with good reason.

Now Father Jonas's whine caught Michael's attention. "I didn't want to discuss this matter at all. It's a dreadful charge to bring against a brother."

Liar! thought Michael. Hypocrite!

The Patriarch waved Jonas to silence. "Yes, we understand. But wait a moment! Your written statement lacks certain facts—namely, when did the alleged offense take place?"

"I knew you were going to ask me that. Um—at first I tried to put it out of my mind. I couldn't believe what I saw. I didn't want to."

Michael snorted. Those nearby frowned at him.

But the judges remained silent, their faces composed and emotionless. Finally, the Bishop of Cyzicus repeated the question. "Indeed, when did this incident take place? You must have some idea."

Jonas wiped his forehead with his faded sleeve. "It was in the spring, I think."

"It was in the spring, to be sure!" Michael said.

Father Zosimas glanced at Michael, but something in the monk's blue eyes shrank.

Now was the time.

"Father Zosimas," said Michael. "Would you please tell the court what you told me?"

Zosimas turned away and bowed his head.

The Bishop of Cyzicus leaned across the table and wagged his finger at Michael. "Sir, hold your peace for now. You'll have your chance to speak."

Though Michael's emotions seethed like the lye in Saponas's factory, he lowered his eyes deferentially. He'd have to be patient for Zosimas's sake. He would not spoil any chance of clearing him.

Instead, Zosimas himself stood up and addressed the judges. "As God is my witness, the incident Father Jonas describes never took place—at least not with myself as one of the participants. I repeat—" He reached into his robes and pulled out his written statement.

The Patriarch nodded. "We know what you wrote. You deny the charge."

"Yes, Your Holiness. I deny all the charges brought against me. Though I'm a sinful man, I've never done what these people accuse me of."

The bishops regarded Zosimas solemnly. "You have nothing else to say?" asked one.

Zosimas waved the document. "It's all here. I am innocent of these offenses."

The Patriarch set down a pen. "The court will adjourn briefly. Afterwards, we'll hear the witnesses for the defendant."

§

During the recess, Michael and Father Zosimas met out in the corridor.

"Michael, you don't look well today," said the latter. "What's wrong?" But Zosimas looked none too well himself. He was pale, with gray circles under his eyes.

Michael felt as though something were stuck in his throat. "Ah—yesterday noon, after the court closed, I went to a wine shop and got drunk."

Zosimas reached up and placed a hand on Michael's shoulder. "I believe that the ancients recommended cabbage for a hangover. That's certainly better than a dose of the same poison." The monk didn't say what he might have said—that he'd never needed to use the remedy himself.

Michael hung his head. "I had only a bread crust."

"I hope it wasn't my predicament that...affected you."

"No." Michael looked him in the eye again. "Or not entirely."

"Oh dear. Then what was it?"

Michael took a deep breath and exhaled slowly. "Yesterday morning, before the court opened, I happened to meet...Barbara."

Zosimas closed his eyes. "Ohhh!"

"I hadn't seen her for years. We talked briefly—about the trial. She's in sympathy with you."

"Indeed? What happened then?"

"Evidently Lady Olympia saw us together. At noon I

sought her out. But she asked questions—about Barbara. What else could I tell her but the truth?"

Zosimas clasped Michael's forearm. "I understand now."

"I know that I have no right to expect anything from her, but now she despises me. She believes that I'm a vile person who amuses himself with loose women."

"Come no. You know that many people believe that men should be as virtuous as they expect women to be. You were brought up that way. So was I. And so, evidently, were Lady Olympia's brothers."

"I know. I can even see the humor in the situation. How many women have confronted their menfolk with such lapses?"

"They should, but usually it's the other way around," said Zosimas.

"Yes, but— Oh, I shouldn't be thinking of myself now!"

"Michael, I'm so sorry!"

Chapter 32

When the court reopened, Michael was pleased to learn that a number of people would testify for Zosimas. He had known about the Abbot of the Studion and Mother Athanasia, but several other monks and laymen had come as well.

First the Abbot spoke, stroking his white beard: he'd known Zosimas for nearly thirty years. Since that time, when Zosimas had entered the monastery, he had always exhibited an honest, open disposition. He had never done anything underhanded, let alone dishonorable. "He told his thoughts to me almost daily, and I've never had any reason to believe that he was troubled by such passions as the plaintiffs accuse him of.

Peter of Serrhes challenged him. "What if he was lying? Of course, he wouldn't tell you!"

"How dare you?" retorted Zosimas's defenders. "Enough!"

"I tell you," said the Abbot, "I observed him myself for all that time. Until the complaints in question were lodged, no one ever said anything against him."

Someone in the back row hooted.

"Silence!" commanded the Patriarch. "Either we'll have order or we'll adjourn."

Michael set his teeth. Was this what the monk's accusers wanted—to wear his supporters down, until they lost either their self-control or their will to fight?

Still, he was glad when a commotion arose in the rear of the hall. Several men were shaking their fists at Peter of

Serrhes, making sure he'd keep his mouth shut.

But Michael did not know how they were going to answer the grocer's charge that Father Zosimas had been lying to the Abbot. How could any mortal man see into another's heart?

The Patriarch, who was surely aware of the problem, did his best. "We'll examine the next witness," he said, "one who's known the defendant all his life. I mean his sister, Mother Anastasia, Abbess of St. Xenia's Convent. She became a nun ten years ago, soon after she was widowed."

"I object!" The people turned to see Peter of Serrhes on his feet. "Get this woman out of here! Women don't belong—"

"Enough!" said the Patriarch. "I see no reason why this *person,* a woman of honorable character, should not testify. Does anyone?"

Nobody answered. Michael assumed that nobody dared to.

Now the Bishop of Cyzicus spoke. "Mother Anastasia, we have your statement here, but we'd like you to tell us about your brother."

The aging nun's blue eyes shone with pride and affection, and the many wrinkles that scored her fair face seemed to vanish. "As you must know, we come from a military family. Our father, a *turmarch,* commanded an army division. I was called Alexandra then. I had two brothers that I hardly knew. They died when I was very small. But I spent much time with my younger brothers. I'm only two years older than Naum, who's now lieutenant-general of the army of the theme, and five years older than

Father Zosimas, who was christened Zenon."

"As a boy, Zenon, was much like any other *turmarch's* son, only better. He liked to ride and practiced archery, but he was also eager to learn reading, writing and numbers. In addition, he was more pious than the rest of us and went to church without fidgeting or complaining."

Father Jonas twisted a strand of his beard around his index finger, then addressed the Patriarch. "How long must we listen to these lies? What sister would testify against her brother? She shouldn't even be here."

Anastasia glowered at him. "A sister who loves the truth more than anything else. I happen to be telling the truth."

"Silence!" warned the Patriarch. "The Lady Abbess may continue."

"Of course, one mustn't have an erroneous impression of Zenon," she said, nodding significantly at Father Jonas. "His disposition was never morbid or sanctimonious. Naum, he, and I often played together—war games, of course. Unfortunately, one of us always had to be a political rebel or a Saracen emir."

"My sister made a very fierce Saracen," said Zosimas.

Smiling, the judges regarded her with interest.

"Zenon was as mischievous as Naum—or any other boy," she continued.

"Really?" inquired one of the bishops. "What did he do?"

"Oh, he teased me, and put crumbs in my bed."

The judges smiled again.

"I retaliated, of course," she said. "Once I caught a frog and put it in *his* bed."

The Patriarch chuckled—a sight new to Michael—while the other judges laughed softly. Soon the whole court was in a mirthful uproar.

When the laughter had all but died away, Father Jonas, cleared his throat noisily. "I daresay we've heard enough of the escapades of the defendant and his hoydenish sister."

The Abbot ignored him. "As you all can see, they're not monsters."

Jonas opened his mouth to reply, but a plainly-dressed man forestalled him. "Your Holiness?"

Zosimas leaned towards Michael. "That fellow was a servant in my sister's house."

"You know," said the servant, "Father Jonas must consider himself the result of a second virgin birth."

The Patriarch glared at him. "See here! We won't countenance blasphemy in this court. And this is a holy place."

The man hung his head. "Sorry! I didn't mean it that way. But ain't it blasphemy if someone thinks so highly of himself?"

Someone in the back hooted.

The Patriarch cast a significant glance at Jonas, then at the servant. "Of course...if anyone did think so highly of himself..."

Michael could not resist a jibe. "Father Jonas doesn't have parents as we do. He was hatched...from a serpent's egg."

"Michael!" Zosimas placed a hand on Michael's shoulder.

The judges struggled to keep their faces straight. "Ah—

we'll hear the rest of the Abbess's testimony," the Patriarch managed to say.

"Now, when I was sixteen," she continued, "I married Alexander Argyros, an officer—a *topoteretes*—in the Excubitors, and came to live here in the Capital. I lost touch with Zenon for a few years."

"In the meantime, he studied with some of the best teachers in the provinces, and exhausted their knowledge by the time he turned fifteen. So, he left our parents' home and joined my household in the City. He was accepted at the School of the Holy Apostles, where he remained until his twentieth year, when he decided to enter the monastery. I had ample opportunity to observe him during that time."

"Forgive me," put in the Bishop of Cyzicus, "but how much could you have known of your brother's habits?"

"Why, I was the lady of the house. Who would know better? My husband spent much of his time on duty at the Palace, or campaigning with the Emperor."

The judges nodded.

"I kept a firm hand on things. And what I couldn't see for myself, I found out by questioning the servants and the grooms. One of them is Elias, the man who just spoke. He can confirm what I've told you."

"Just what did you learn by observing your brother's conduct?" the Bishop asked.

"I never had any reason to believe he...liked men, but he did notice girls. He often spoke to them when we were out in the marketplace. But he was always respectful. And he didn't pursue that...interest."

Somebody sniggered, but the Patriarch shot him a

withering glance.

"I know well," said the Abbess, "that if he'd wished, he would have been a great statesman, or a scholar. He could have found himself a good and noble wife. However, he preferred a higher life. If he took a vow of chastity, he kept it, and that is that. He was a virgin!"

Peter guffawed.

"*Was* perhaps, "said Jonas, sniffing. "We were all born that way."

Michael recoiled, as if from a kick in the stomach. He jumped up, shaking his fist at the monk. "Why you—"

"Calm yourself, Michael," said the Patriarch. "I promise—we'll hear you next."

The Abbess took a deep breath. Her eyes were moist. "I know—he still is."

Peter of Serrhes made a rude noise. "Oh, get rid of this old hag!"

The ancient nun sitting next to the Abbess all but spat. "This young whelp needs a few swats on the backside."

Mother Anastasia didn't bother to reproach her. She merely wiped her eyes on her sleeve and patted the crone's forearm.

"And as for Father Jonas," said the latter, "he reminds me of a nasty little boy in our apartment block, when I was a child. When my sister and I played in the courtyard, he'd drop turds from his balcony."

"That's enough," said the Abbess, patting the old nun's faded sleeve. "We understand."

"Quiet, all of you!" The Patriarch grimaced, closing his nostrils. He looked as though Jonas had indeed brought "turds" into court.

Gradually, the racket subsided. Then, to everyone's astonishment, the Novice Matthew tottered to his feet. As a murmur filled the chapel, he stifled a choking sound. "Please... Your Holiness...may I go out?"

"Go ahead."

Matthew closed the doors behind him. But through them, everyone could hear the spasmodic croaks of his retching.

Michael wondered if this were a performance, like the novice's fainting spell yesterday, meant to elicit people's sympathy. But he rather doubted it. Both episodes seemed very real.

The Patriarch held his peace until Matthew returned, wiping his mouth with a handkerchief.

"Now," he said, glancing at Michael, "we will hear the testimony of Michael Taronites, an agent of the Post."

Michael looked down at his boots and felt his ears burn.

"As all of you surely know, Taronites is a hero of the Empire. He uncovered a nefarious plot to kill the Emperor and put a usurper on the throne. Now, he has known Father Zosimas for most of his life—"

"I object!" Peter of Serrhes stood up. "Yesterday morning, before the court opened, this ruffian beat up a man and cursed him out with the foulest language."

"We've heard that accusation already," said the Patriarch.

Now the Abbot of the Studion spoke up. "I repeat—he'd been provoked. Some ne'er-do-well crudely insulted the defendant and his sister. And though Tarnonites did call

261

him a regrettable name, I'm sure we've all heard worse. Few of us have led completely sheltered lives." He glanced at Father Jonas.

"Do you condone violence?" asked the latter.

"Of course not," replied the Abbot. "It's hardly the preferred method of righting wrongs. But, as I said before, it's understandable under the circumstances. Taronites couldn't just stand there and let his friends be slandered, could he? He only punched the man in the nose and—er—offered him his handkerchief afterwards."

"Ahem!" said the Patriarch. "This court has no choice but to consider Taronites as an acceptable witness for Father Zosimas, as a Christian in good standing."

"Wait!" put in Peter of Serrhes. "Wasn't there a scandal at the Palace a few years ago? Something about some women?"

So! Michael considered what had been in the back of his mind. If he had slept with the Augusta's maid, he could be accused of immorality and barred as a witness. Now he knew for certain that Saponas had orchestrated that incident, and that he was working with the odious Peter of Serrhes.

"If there was a scandal," countered the Patriarch, "it occurred many years ago. It is past, and the witness is a man of flawless reputation... Now, Taronites, would you like to tell us about your acquaintance with the defendant?"

Actually, Michael wished to discuss another matter entirely, but he thought it wise to comply—at least long enough to catch the accusers off guard.

He stood. "I've known Father Zosimas almost all my

life," he began. "Long before I was born, he was my father's friend. They attended the School of the Holy Apostles together."

Father Jonas shook a bony finger at him, then turned to the judges. "See? Taronites cannot be an unbiased witness. The monk was a family friend. And what sort of relationship did he have with the witness's father?"

Michael dug his nails into his palms. What he'd been planning to do made more and more sense.

Now Elias the servant stood up. "Will someone shut the mouth of that smarmy little snake? Or we can settle this outside."

"Order!" said the Patriarch. "Such charges are without foundation. We'll hear out Taronites."

Peter of Serrhes made a catcall, but the Patriarch waved him to silence. "Michael's father Theodore—may God rest his soul—was a man of good repute. And he defended the Empress in a very dark time."

"That's true," said Michael. "And as for Father Zosimas, he always spoke of him as a high moral example. He wanted Zosimas to be my spiritual father."

Michael felt a twinge of sorrow. He had already lost his father. Would he now lose Zosimas? "Throughout my boyhood, I always thought of Father Zosimas as the epitome of virtue...and of kindness." He swallowed the lump in his throat and glared at Father Jonas, who was *not* kind. "For this reason I find the charges against Father Zosimas appalling. For this reason I *know* that the plaintiffs have some vile ulterior motive."

He then turned to Peter. "I'm surprised you didn't bring

your cousin today—if he really is your cousin. Actually, you have no business in this court without him."

Peter's gray eyes widened. "Well, of course he's my cousin."

Michael nodded in satisfaction. Those seated behind him began to whisper. He continued: "Where is Luke, anyway?"

"At home. He's sick."

"Oh, really? The novice Matthew isn't well, and he still came today."

Michael looked around the chapel. "I wonder if Luke is anything he says he is. I want him brought back here. Do you know what I plan to do with him then?"

Peter's broad face blanched. "N-no."

Michael couldn't resist a smirk. No doubt the wretch was thinking of torture or castration.

"I'll tell the whole court now, in detail." The more Michael drew things out, the more Peter would squirm—and, hopefully, lose his composure. "I'll pull off the rascal's boots and examine his feet. If he really is a shepherd boy and not a shopkeeper or an idle catamite, he'll have calluses an inch thick."

Some of the judges gasped, and Peter let out a groan. His face turned an apoplectic red.

Behind Michael, a cheer went up.

"Well done!" said the Bishop of Cyzicus.

"We need to bring the boy back here," said the Patriarch.

Michael addressed the judges. "But there's more, much more that's amiss with our accusers. Take the case of Father Jonas."

Someone audibly drew a breath.

"Earlier I asked Father Zosimas to tell the court what he told me about Father Jonas. But I fear he won't do it."

Zosimas, he noticed, had buried his face in his hands.

"I'm sorry, Father, but the truth must be told. It's for your own good."

Michael took a deep breath and faced the judges again. "Father Zosimas is keeping silent out of the goodness of his heart. He's forgiven the offender, so why, according to his understanding, should anybody else know?"

"Please," the Patriarch put in," forgiven him for what? To what are you referring?"

"Father Jonas has given you a distorted version of the episode in question," Michael replied. "This is what really happened on that night last spring. Father Jonas approached the defendant after Compline and arranged to meet him behind the scriptorium, supposedly to discuss some urgent matter. When the defendant, thinking no evil, kept the appointment, the plaintiff made indecent advances to him. The defendant fled and never told a soul besides me."

§

On account of the commotion following Michael's revelation, the Patriarch adjourned court for the day. Peter of Serrhes, Father Jonas, Matthew, and their sympathizers promptly made for the door, but Michael, encouraged by the turn of events, hung back to wait for Zosimas's party.

"Don't you want to get something to eat or drink?" the monk asked Michael.

"I feel better, and I need some fresh air most of all."

"What was wrong with Matthew?" one of the group

asked Michael.

"I have a good idea." But it was too soon to explain.

As soon as they descended the front steps of the Patriarchate, a cheering throng pressed towards them. "What happened?" people asked, tugging on their sleeves. "Has he been cleared?"

"Not yet," said Michael. "But God willing, we'll clear him soon. We've made a breach in their fortifications."

The throng waved, and sent up a cheer. As many as could, men and women alike, pushed forward to kiss Zosimas's hand and exchange bear hugs with Michael.

Off to one side Mother Anastasia and the nuns were chanting: "He hath shown strength with His arm. He hath scattered the proud in the imagination of their heart."

Michael cautioned the people. "I repeat: there's been no decision yet. But now we have a chance."

"Yes, we do," said Zosimas, who was momentarily unencumbered by admirers. He smiled faintly.

But his smile quickly vanished. "Michael, look over there—by the Milion Arch! That man—I've seen him before!"

Michael followed the monk's gaze. Several men stood near the gold-domed structure, but Michael knew exactly which one Zosimas meant. He was tall and broad-shouldered, in a fur hat and a plain, dark-colored cloak. A flowing white beard complemented his grave, austere face.

He was the man Michael had seen leaving Peter's store, the one that the grocer and his wife had called Boian.

Chapter 33

Even as Michael and Father Zosimas gazed after Boian, the old man receded into the crowd, then vanished completely.

"We'll never catch up with him now," said Michael. A jostling, boisterous crowd clogged the pavement between the Patriarchate and the Milion Arch.

"Who is he, anyway?"

"I've heard him called Boian—he was in the back room of the grocery with Peter and his wife last Friday morning—and I saw him leave afterwards." Michael cast a significant glance at Zosimas. "Where have you seen him?"

"In the monastery church. It was over a month ago. I think he came more than once...Boian, eh? His name means 'warlike.'"

"He's the one! He must have threatened Matthew and induced him to accuse you. Maybe he even influenced Father Jonas. He must be working with Peter of Serrhes, and we'll find out who else."

§

Meanwhile, Father Jonas, the novice Matthew, and their supporters made their way back to the Studion. They had passed through the Forum of Constantine and were now crossing the Forum of Theodosius, the next square westward on the Mese.

"Wh-what happened to Peter anyway," asked Matthew, clenching the reins of his horse.

Jonas brushed aside a strand of lank, greasy hair that had escaped from beneath his cap. "He said he was going back to the store. He was needed there. What of it?"

"Nothing." Matthew swallowed hard. He pulled a grimy handkerchief from his robes and dabbed at his mouth with it. "Oh, my God! Oh, my God!"

"What's wrong with you, anyway? I don't believe what I'm hearing. You're taking the name of God in vain."

Matthew did not reply. Only then did Father Jonas realize that the youth, far from blaspheming, had uttered an anguished prayer.

"Don't you realize the gravity of our situation," said Father Jonas. "If he's found innocent..."

Matthew made a choking sound. "I know."

"You're the one who...involved me," said Father Jonas. "I'd heard those rumors you'd been spreading and thought—"

Matthew groaned, and began to weep, but he was composed enough to throw away his messy handkerchief and wipe his eyes and nose on his sleeve. "What did you expect me to do under those circumstances? Here I was, a youth who knew nothing of the world. I was scandalized by what I saw in the scriptorium. It wasn't enough for me to take my complaint to the Abbot. I felt abandoned. I wanted company."

"That's just what I thought." Jonas urged his mount into a trot as they passed through a marble arch, leaving the forum behind. He bowed his head in thought, then narrowed his eyes knowingly. "Tell me, my son, why did you really do it?"

Matthew puffed out his chest. "It's just as I said. Father Zosimas..."

Shrugging, Father Jonas let his reins drop. "If you say so."

"There's nothing more to tell... Oh, excuse me, I—"

But Jonas heard an ominous hiss, not retching.

"Ohhh!"

"Matthew, what?" Father Jonas turned. For some reason he was not surprised to see an arrow vibrating in the novice's chest.

§

Less than a quarter of an hour later, Father Zosimas's party emerged from the Forum of Theodosius: an odd assembly of militiamen and monks blocked their way.

The monks, thought, Michael, looked quite familiar; yes, it was *those* monks, those with Father Jonas.

Michael slipped out of the saddle. "What's going on here?"

Turning, Father Jonas wiped a lank strand of hair from his eyes. He looked even paler than usual. "So, it's you!" he remarked.

Then his outrage dissolved into a groan. "Matthew's been shot." He stepped aside.

A semicircle had formed around a human shape on the cobblestones.

"Indeed," Michael whispered, as he approached the supine figure. Matthew's clear-skinned, sparsely-bearded face was comely, even in death. Though his eyes had been closed, an arrow still protruded from his chest. There were no identifying marks on the shaft—only a place where something had been scraped off.

"Quickly!" Michael averted his eyes from the body and

269

addressed one of the police. "Have you—"

The militiaman nodded, clutching the truncheon at his belt. With his free hand he gestured behind him. "We've sent someone to search the houses up there."

"Good! I'm from the Post myself, and this incident may concern us as well of you. There's more taking place than meets the eye. We'd like a copy of your records of this incident, and the arrow as evidence."

"The Post? As far as I'm concerned, you can have whatever you want, but you'll have to talk to my superior first."

Michael heard his companions ride up behind him, and turned towards them. "The novice Matthew has been murdered."

Groaning loudly, they crossed themselves, as did Jonas's party.

But within moments they had all recuperated enough to glare at each other—all but Zosimas, who dismounted and came forward. "Well, God rest his soul."

Father Jonas shot him a hateful glance.

Michael couldn't resist a jab. "Father couldn't have done it. We were well behind you."

"Who could have, then?" demanded one of Jonas's companions. "What harm did he ever do—"

"Matthew tried to do much harm to Father Zosimas here." Michael laid a hand on the latter's forearm. "But I believe that somebody forced him."

"Forced him? To do what?" replied Jonas.

"To bring a false accusation. You saw how ill he was, both yesterday and today."

Jonas's tone was uncertain. "Yes."

"He was about to break," said Michael. "That's why they had to kill him."

"*They?* Who do you mean?"

"Do you really not know? Where's Peter of Serrhes, anyway?"

Jonas sucked in his breath.

"In any case, the truth will soon come out." Michael would let them think he knew more than he did.

But he had other concerns now as well. "I'm going to inform the Palace," he said, swinging back into the saddle. He was about to wheel his mount around when he had another idea. "Perhaps you should come with me," he told Zosimas, "in case I run across Boian again."

§

After the midday meal, Irene Macrembolitissa, Olympia's mother, followed her husband into his study. She gazed uneasily at his broad back. "Dear…"

Basil Macrembolites shoved a few parchment scraps and an ink pot into the side compartment of his desk, then whirled around. "Please! I have to tidy up before he gets here."

Irene crossed the carpet to him. Placing her hand on his arm, she looked him straight in the eye; her height gave her some advantage. "I wish you'd reconsider. Or at least, don't rush into it."

His heavy, graying eyebrows drew together. "Come now, woman! You sound like Acropolites."

"That's what he told you? There! You see?"

"I'll make no commitments. Today I'll simply talk to the

man."

"Good! You know nothing about him, anyway."

"Only that he's a judge, and that he has money, and properties both here in the City and in Bithynia."

Irene sniffed.

Basil raised his voice. "Listen!" His face darkened. "We have to act now, while Olympia has some reputation left. After that overnight expedition to the widow's—"

"Acropolites said that she was well chaperoned. Do you think he lied?"

"I know he didn't. And our people vouched for her."

"Why are you concerned then?"

"Because people talk. Also, because she didn't even ask me. She should do only what I wish her to do. I should send her to a nunnery."

"She might not object to that... Alas, I understand you now."

"Good! I lay down the law in my house... And about Acropolites, he's a eunuch. What does he know?"

"He knows her well."

Basil waved his wife to silence. "He doesn't want to lose her."

§

Olympia paced her third-floor bedroom. How many times since she'd come up had she gone from the windows to her dressing table, then back again?

Though she'd slept badly after yesterday's distressing events, she'd gone to Acropolites's office anyway. But once there, she felt so weary that she'd asked for the rest of the day off.

272

Alas, how could she rest, when she was being sold like a cow? She might as well go back to her teacher's. There at least she'd be able to do something besides wring her hands in regret.

She had been shrewish to Michael, but she had been greatly scandalized. She had thought him above such behavior, but now she realized that she should have been prepared for this disappointment. Several years ago, when *Michael Taronites* was only a name to her, she had heard rumors about his involvement in some matter considered unsuitable for the ears of a proper young lady. But then again, much that took place in the Palace was not fit for the ears of a proper young lady.

And now she had learned the truth, or at least his account of it. Should she believe him?

Now a faint murmur reached her from the window, drawing her back to it. Through the small panes, she could make out two men down in the garden. Their backs to her, they walked towards the fountain. She recognized her father's stocky form, but not the other's slender build.

She scowled. That must be the suitor.

Her father hoped—indeed he expected—that she would watch from the window. Well, here she was, and so far, her opinion was unfavorable. She could not distinguish the man's features from this distance, but she could see that he was tall. And he walked with the measured gait of a mature man. When he spoke, he inclined his head only slightly and gestured with fluttering hands. There was a certain preciousness, a fussiness, about him.

Ugh! She quickly looked away. She did not want to be

mated with a stranger, like a beast in the barnyard.

Her elder sister Elizabeth often taunted her about such feelings, with a bluntness that would have horrified their parents. Bawdy talk was her way of asserting herself—along with her import business—just as medicine was Olympia's.

"What are you afraid of?" Elizabeth would ask. "You're the doctor here. You ought to know that no one ever died of it. In fact—"

Elizabeth's argument was poorly chosen. Not a few women died in childbirth, though obviously Elizabeth had not. So far she had two children.

But it was not the fear of pain and death that had put Olympia off marriage. It was her sense of purpose: she knew she must be a physician. Still, she knew that eventually she would have to conform to the demands of society: she'd either marry or retire to a nunnery. The latter alternative looked more and more attractive.

She thought of her sister's jibes; yes, she was a doctor. But all she knew of the relations between men and women she had learned from medical texts. When had she ever been troubled by lust?

But she understood that she was not being completely honest with herself. She caught her breath as the warm tide of realization swept over her. There was a man she wanted, and she was jealous of *that woman*, who had once possessed him.

Even so, she thought, lust was hardly worth the energy expended in satisfying it. Eventually even the happiest married couples tired of each other and took each other for granted—when they weren't screeching at each other like fishmongers. Her parents did as much. Just this noon, her father had been yelling at her mother again.

Finally, a thought, a small comfort, came to her.

She gazed into her silver mirror and wiped a tear from her cheek. "So," she told herself. "You're not only an angel of mercy but a human being after all."

Chapter 34

Back at the Post, Michael settled Father Zosimas in his tiny office, then dashed off to consult with the Commander of the Varangians. "I tell you—the two cases are connected," he said.

The Akoluthos managed a stiff-lipped smile. "So you've said."

"I'm right. You'll see." So he felt, though he still had no proof.

He then asked the Varangian to question anew all those under suspicion for Bourtzes's murder: Saponas, Syropoulos, Tripsychos, Blachernites—the Logothete of the Dromos. "And—yes—interrogate Metiga the Patzinak, even if you have to drag him from whatever tavern, whatever bordello, in whatever sort of stupor."

Michael also warned the Akoluthos to maintain contact with the militia, who would inform him if they found anyone answering to Boian's description. And the militia, for their part, would interrogate Peter of Serrhes: did he truly go back to his store after the church court was dismissed?

Once Michael's plans were laid, he returned to his office and perched on a stool in the corner; Zosimas occupied his desk chair.

"I'll wager that Boian is a Bogomil perfect," Michael said. He rested his elbows on his knees, his face in his hands.

"Games of chance are never prudent."

Michael looked up and saw a twinkle in Zosimas's eye.

"That was a figure of speech, as well you know. Don't you think it's likely?"

"Yes. As you say, he must have threatened poor Matthew—may God rest his soul."

Michael stared at the monk's mild countenance. "I can't quite forgive him. I'm surprised you—"

"I try. He must have repented of his accusation. You saw how dreadful he looked."

Michael scowled. "Yes, but still— Well, I wonder what Boian threatened him with. He must be the culprit. But is he the ringleader of the group?"

Sighing, Father Zosimas rubbed his eyes; the whites looked cloudy with fatigue. "He may have attained to the Bogomils' perverted standards of perfection. He may even lead their prayer meetings. But that doesn't necessarily make him a good administrator."

"No, but a man of his demeanor could strike fear into anyone. Still, I doubt he killed Matthew. We were far behind the novice and his friends when we saw Boian at the Milion. Only if he were a magician as well as a perfect could he have reached the Forum of Theodosius so quickly."

Zosimas chuckled.

"It's more likely that Peter killed the novice," Michael continued. "He as well as Boian could be the instigator of the plot against you. And if not he, then one or our—ah— friends in the Palace."

"God willing, we'll soon learn who." Zosimas folded his hands in his lap.

Mere minutes later, someone rapped on the door.

Michael jumped up. Perhaps now they'd know. "Yes?

Come in."

Askold Sviatoslavich, the stocky Varangian who had helped Michael in his first investigation, strode in. "We—" Seeing Father Zosimas, he startled. "Ah! Why, you must be—I didn't expect to find you here." He kissed Zosimas's hand, then addressed Michael. "We have news for you. Peter of Serrhes is in his store, and claims he went straight back this noon. His wife and cousin Luke can vouch for him. So far, the militia have found no sign of Boian, and our people have yet to find Metiga."

Michael sighed in exasperation.

"Also," said Askold, "Syropoulos has been on the Palace grounds all morning—many have seen him—and he dined with the Emperor this noon. The Logothete of the Dromos has a similar alibi, and also dined with His Majesty."

Michael snorted. "That means nothing in itself. They could have hired someone."

"And Tripsychos didn't come in at all today. He sent word that he was ill."

"We'll check on that." But now Michael noticed that the Varangian's eyes burned with eagerness. "Yes? What else?"

"Saponas has been gone since early morning. He set out on horseback, equipped with a bow and quiver. He said he was going hunting in the hills north of the City."

Chapter 35

"So!" Michael's pulse quickened. "Did Saponas in fact leave the City?" He thought of the arrow in Matthew's chest. The identifying mark had been scraped off the shaft, but previously it could have borne the same black band that Michael had seen on those in Saponas's Palace apartments.

"I want the guards at the gates questioned about his comings and goings, and as soon as he turns up—"

"We should arrest him," said Askold. "But do you think that he will come back to the City, sir, if he's left?"

"If he's innocent, he'll return. If not, he might well come back anyway, to appear so. In any case, arrest him."

"Yes, sir."

"And there's something else we need. You, or one of your comrades, should contact the militia. Have them find out if anyone caught sight of Saponas near the Forum of Theodosius this noon."

"Done," said Askold, and went on his way.

Now Zosimas spoke. "Do you think Saponas is the culprit?"

Michael began to pace the floor. "I believe that someone killed Matthew to silence him, somebody plotting against you. He might well be behind this plot to discredit you—if he is indeed a Bogomil. I don't know what relationship he has to Peter of Serrhes and his so-called cousin."

"I see."

"Evidently, he knows how to shoot. He could have been the sniper last Friday morning. He doesn't have a good alibi for that time or for the night of Bourtzes's death. On the other hand, none of our other suspects have been cleared."

"If Saponas does return...or if he's caught..."

"Then we'll question him, of course."

"Er—of course." Zosimas bowed his head and appeared to be contemplating something unpleasant.

An uneasy silence hung between them. Michael felt relieved when a knock on the door broke it. "Yes?" He stopped his pacing.

The door swung open, and the trim form of the Logothete of the Dromos appeared on the threshold. "Taronites, you wanted to see me?"

Michael swallowed his embarrassment. "Ah—the Varangians told me what I needed to know."

"Yes, I've been here all morning." The Logothete's white, bushy eyebrows drew together when he noticed Father Zosimas, sitting at Michael's desk. "Ah, so you're—" he muttered. He made no move to receive Zosimas's blessing.

Michael understood, and glowered at his superior.

A scowl crossed Blachernites's face. "If there's nothing more you need to know, I'll be going. It's time I was back at my desk."

When the Logothete had gone, Michael turned back to Zosimas. "I'm sorry he was so rude to you. Either he believes all that rubbish—or he invented it."

"Come now, Michael. You don't know that for a fact."

"What I do know is that he's not kindly disposed to you, *and* that he can't prove his whereabouts at the time of Bourtzes's death. And I haven't forgotten that he was one

280

of the three people—aside from the Emperor—at that meeting where Bourtzes's mission was discussed."

"I see. God willing, the whole affair will be settled soon."

Michael didn't see how. In his desperation, he felt an aching hollow in the pit of his stomach and realized that he had eaten nothing all day, except for that crust of bread early this morning. And his hangover had mysteriously vanished. And the poor monk—when had he eaten? "I don't know when it will be over," he said. "So, for the present, let's try to find some food."

§

After a meal of bread, olives, and watered wine—obtained from one of the Palace's many kitchens—Michael and Father Zosimas parted company on the walk behind the Post. "I need some time alone, to pray," said the latter. "If you need me, I'll be in the Church of the Mother of God."

Michael watched Zosimas's compact, sturdy figure recede down the steps and across the mosaic courtyard. The deepening shadows of late afternoon obscured both the images on the pavement and the bulk of the three churches that rose behind it.

Finally, the monk disappeared into the atrium of the central church, The Mother of God of the Lighthouse, and Michael returned to his office. Despite the gathering dusk, he did not light a lamp but sat down at his desk, yawning, involuntarily. His head felt unbearably heavy, and he rested it on the desk. Sleep enveloped him almost immediately.

It seemed only minutes later that someone seized his shoulders and shook him awake. "Come on, Taronites, we got the bastard."

A Varangian! Michael groaned and sat up, rubbing his eyes. The room lay in darkness. Only a dim light spilled on from the corridor. "Who?" he asked.

"Saponas."

Saponas! Michael looked up at the red-tunicked guard, one he knew only by sight. "Did he—"

"He came back by himself. Let's go."

Outside, naked tree branches waved in the wind. The hanging lanterns flickered. When Michael and his companion turned onto a narrow path between dark, formless shrubs, Michael felt a chill sweat run down his back. Did he hear someone behind him, padding over the dry grass? Last Thursday night, when he'd walked here, he was certain he'd been followed.

Even though he had an armed Varangian with him, he was glad when they reached the glowing light of a columned gallery and gladder still when they crossed the Guards' courts and entered the Varangians' headquarters. Here lamps blazed, and armed soldiers rushed back and forth.

Michael and the Guard passed the office of the Akoluthos, stopping only at the far end of the hallway. The Varangian knocked on a heavy planked door and called out. "He's here, sir!"

Inside, someone grunted in assent, then threw the door open.

The room behind it had stark, whitish walls. Michael went in and immediately recoiled from the bright light and heat. To one side, a rack of lamps burned. At the back of the room stood a brazier filled with glowing coals.

But Michael quickly accustomed himself to his surroundings. Saponas, he saw, was slumped on a stool near the center of the room. Several Varangians flanked him.

The buffoon managed a grin. "Well, they've sent me an archangel."

Michael ignored the jibe. "So," he began, "do you know why you're here?"

Saponas shrugged. "I know only what they've told me."

Michael turned toward the Akoluthos, who sat at a table near the lamps. "What has he confessed?"

"Nothing." The Varangian grimaced.

"Have you had a report from the walls yet?" asked Michael. "Did Saponas actually leave the City this morning? And if so, when did he come back?"

"We don't know yet," said the Akoluthos, rubbing his close-cropped beard. "And we haven't heard from the militia, either."

"May I question the prisoner now?"

"Go ahead. But so far, this interrogation has gone nowhere. I think we ought to try another method."

"There's no need for that," said Michael.

Breathing noisily, Saponas shifted his position on the stool. Michael thought that he was no longer his usual merry self.

He began his questioning, but with an inexplicable lump of dread in the pit of his stomach. "You left the Palace early this morning?"

Michael studied Saponas's clothing: a plain tunic, coarse wool breeches and hose, boots. The man's story was quite plausible. "So, what did you bag?"

Saponas flinched and licked his lips. They appeared to shrivel before Michael's eyes. "Nothing."

"That's right," said the Akoluthos. "He came back empty-handed."

Michael addressed the prisoner. "You must not have tried very hard...if you were out there all day."

"I'm out of practice. This is the first time I've been in a long time."

"Oh? Michael turned to the Akoluthos. "Do you have his equipment? I'd like a look at one of his arrows."

One of the Varangians rummaged around in a box and pulled out a shaft. Michael recognized the black band. "Yes—just as I remembered. Did he have any that were unmarked, or with the band scraped off?"

"No."

"If he did, he threw them away," Michael concluded. "Matthew was killed by an arrow with the owner's mark scraped off—a mark in the same position as this one," he added, tapping the shaft.

Saponas snorted. "It could have been anybody's. Why mine?"

"Because you were near the Forum of Theodosius this noon," Michael replied. He had no proof, but shock tactics might work. "And you can't account for your activities last Friday morning, when someone shot at me near Peter's grocery."

Michael watched Saponas; did he react at all? No, not even to Peter's name.

"I went home to look in on my son, and the factory."

"You didn't stay very long," said Michael. "And you

can't account for your actions at an even more critical time."

Saponas emitted a strained laugh. "What are you talking about?"

"Your whereabouts last Monday night."

"Ah—I told you. It's a private matter."

"So, what's the lady's name?"

"I can't say."

Michael thundered at him. "How do you expect us to believe you? How do you expect us to believe that you didn't kill Bourtzes when you were one of the three officials know knew about his mission? How do you expect us to believe that you didn't kill him when you've been plotting against Father Zosimas?"

"Father Zosimas?" Saponas jumped up. Immediately the guards grabbed his shoulders and forced him down again. "That's ridiculous! Why should I have anything to do with him?"

"Father Zosimas's case and Bourtzes's case are connected," said Michael, then paused. *Connected, but how?* So his inner voice prompted him. "You wanted, Matthew dead, and I know why."

Saponas gulped.

Muffled exclamations filled the room. The Akoluthos cleared his throat. "One way or the other, we'll have the truth." He glanced significantly at the men flanking Saponas.

Saponas sputtered. "Wh—why would I want to kill some nonentity of a novice?" he asked, swallowing hard.

"He testified against Father Zosimas," said Michael, "but I believe someone forced him to—perhaps you? His testimony was a lie, and he was about to break. He was visibly ill during the proceedings of the church court. Now, I don't know precisely why you want to discredit Father Zosimas, but suppose you were a Bogomil..."

Saponas laughed. "I, a Bogomil? They don't eat meat, drink wine, or have women. Why would I want to be *that?*"

Michael narrowed his eyes. "On the contrary, the Bogomils have rather...flexible attitudes towards those activities. As I understand, only the Perfect—like your friend Boian—are required to abstain entirely from them."

Saponas pulled out a handkerchief and loudly blew his nose. "Boian? I don't know any Boian!"

"Don't lie as the Bogomils do, whenever it's to their advantage."

"I tell you..."

Gradually Michael became aware of a stirring out in the corridor. Someone rapped on the door and called out in Norse."

"Come in," said the Akoluthos.

A lanky Varangian with a scar on his left cheek strode in and saluted the commander. "Sir, the militia have found no trace of the outlander known as Boian. But Saponas was seen leaving the City through the Blachernae Gate at the first hour of the day. Sometime before noon, he re-entered the City at the Gate of Charisius."

Michael groaned. An inexplicable sorrow possessed him. "So, you killed Matthew...and Bourtzes too."

"No!"

The Akoluthos raised a restraining hand. "Taronites, you're too much the gentleman. At this rate, we'll be here all month."

The guards holding Saponas tightened their grip.

"From now on we'll conduct this interrogation differently," said the Akoluthos, nodding towards the brazier. "Waldemar, heat up that poker."

The scar-faced newcomer approached the live coals.

Blanching, Saponas struggled against his captors. He tried to stand. "No! For God's sake, no!"

Michael turned to the commander. "I'll get him to talk without that. It's stupid to torture a suspect, because he'll tell you whatever you want to hear. He won't—"

"Oh, don't be an old woman! If this doesn't work, we'll take him downstairs."

While two Varangians held Saponas, a third planted a kick in his stomach. "Are you going to tell now, you bastard, you stinking sack of shit?"

Saponas groaned. Michael turned way, but heard something splash on the floor. Then, cringing, he watched out of the corner of his eye as a guard pulled a clump of hair from the prisoner's unkempt beard. An inhuman shriek shook the walls of the room.

Michael sensed charcoal fumes, hot metal, and something worse. His ears began to buzz. He must find a seat before he keeled over.

Someone pushed a stool under him, and he crumpled onto it. Slowly the pounding waves in his head subsided—only to be replaced by a cacophony of protests, shouts, and crashes outside.

Then the door swung open again, thudding against the wall. Someone stepped into the room.

His voice was well-modulated and quite familiar: "Take your hands off him at once!"

Chapter 36

"What in damnation—"

"Oh, crap!"

The guards shouted.

Astonished, Michael jumped up. The room seemed to roll and pitch before his eyes. Minutes passed before he could move.

Finally, he looked towards the doorway. There, through the mist of weakness veiling his eyes, he saw a welcome figure.

He blinked. No, truly he wasn't seeing things.

Bareheaded, a strand of wavy grayish hair stuck to his forehead, Father Zosimas stood just inside the room. His blue eyes, fixed on Saponas, blazed with zeal. "Let him go!"

The Varangians holding Saponas grumbled, but released him. The prisoner rustled his garments, and emitted a low groan.

Now Zosimas shifted his gaze to the back of the room, where Waldemar was holding the poker. "And you—put that thing down."

Somehow the monk had assumed authority here.

And Michael had recovered himself enough to speak. "Father, how did you… What—"

The Akolouthos, who had remained in possession of himself, glared at Zosimas. "What are you doing in my interrogation room?"

"You needn't worry that it was easy to get in. Your men tried to stop me."

The commander grunted and crossed his arms on his

chest.

Michael ignored him and turned to Zosimas. Something else concerned him more. "How did you..." *How did you know to come in time?*

Zosimas advanced into the room, throwing his mantle back over his shoulders. "Why, Michael, I was concerned when you didn't come to the church for me. So I left on my own and headed towards your office. I saw you leaving with a Varangian, and I followed you."

"I see." Michael recalled now that he thought someone was tracking them. "So it was you!"

"Yes. I reached here later and heard the news from another guard. And when the Varangians wouldn't let me in," he added, his eyes now twinkling, "I concluded that my presence might be necessary and elbowed my way to here."

The Akolouthos strode toward him. "You're obstructing an investigation. I ought to—"

But really, Michael wondered, what could the Varangian do? Seize an innocent man, an unarmed monk, and throw him out? Torture him? He could, but the whole world would consider him a monster.

For a moment, though, the Akoluthos stood his ground. "Well, monk, what do you have to say for yourself?"

"I cannot countenance torture and violence."

Now the scar-faced Waldemar broke in. "Listen! We do this for your sake! This scum Saponas killed someone, but he also—"

The Akoluthos scowled at his man. "Don't speak out of turn. We'll see what Saponas did." He cocked an eyebrow at Zosimas. "Yes, we're seeking justice for you. We think that

Saponas killed Matthew so he wouldn't talk. We think Saponas is behind all the slanders."

Zosimas took a resolute step towards the commander. He had to tilt his head back to look the Varangian in the eye. "I wish only to be cleared."

The Akoluthos looked puzzled. "But what—"

"I'm not out for revenge," said Zosimas, "and I don't want to see the prisoner suffer."

The Akoluthos swore under his breath. Then a hush fell upon the room, lasting for several minutes. Finally Saponas groaned again; the patch of raw flesh on his cheek made Michael shudder. But before he could look away, he saw a blank, utterly dumbfounded expression cross the soapmaker's broad face.

Michael swallowed a lump of guilt. Though torture sickened him, he wanted to see Zosimas's accusers pay. If their fate were in his hands, he'd deal with him at the very least as he had dealt with that wretch in front of the Patriarchate.

The Akoluthos, as though guessing Michael's thoughts, shook a finger at Zosimas. "Father, those who choose to live outside the law lose the law's protection and are liable to punishment."

"Yes, but…"

Michael nodded. The Akoluthos had expressed the attitude that he, as a government official, was bound to uphold—just as Michael was. Still, like Zosimas, Michael saw the limitations of this position.

"Consider," he said, as he settled the monk on his stool. "Our purpose now is to uncover the truth. Will torturing the prisoner really help us do so?" Yet most people paid lip service to the belief that torture worked. But he was reluctant to accept it—perhaps because he had once been on the wrong side of the law.

Did torture actually work? That was the point he needed to make now, though he feared that the Akoluthos had little use for philosophical speculation.

"We're not old women or monks," the latter said—even now. "We'll do whatever we have to do to find the truth. So far, we've questioned him politely and learned nothing."

"Think!" Michael retorted. "If he's guilty, he just might confess under torture, but if he's innocent, he'll most probably confess anyway—just to stop the pain. In that case, you'll never have the truth, and the real culprit will escape your hand."

Now Father Zosimas broke in. "What's more; it's wanton cruelty. It's savagery!"

The Akoluthos clutched his close-cropped hair and groaned. "Oh, but monks are a damned nuisance and a pain in the arse!"

"Your language, sir," said Michael. "There's a monk present." Zosimas, he noticed, was sitting unperturbed.

The commander faced the monk. "Er—I'm sorry," he said, then addressed Michael. "So! How do you suggest we question him?"

Michael didn't know. Who did? Once more his gaze fell on the corpulent Saponas, slumped on his seat. Blood, vomit, and mucus stained his tunic.

Michael felt sorry for him, but he knew he had to do his job. "I think the prisoner will be willing to conduct a rational discussion in his present condition."

"What about it, Saponas?" demanded the Akoluthos. "Are you going to talk?"

Saponas raised his shaggy head. His gray eyes looked cloudy with tears, as well as with the traces of debauchery. "Ouch—I don't know," he croaked. "May I have a drink?"

The commander slammed his fist on the table. "We'll have none of your foolery!"

"This is not foolery," said Zosimas, now standing. "Let him clean up, and give him some water."

Most likely not, Michael thought, the drink Saponas had in mind.

One of the guards went out, returning with reinforcements as well as a basin, a linen cloth, a cup, and a pitcher.

Saponas wet the cloth and washed, wincing as the water touched his raw flesh. When he was done, he wadded up the reddened linen and tossed it on the floor. Zosimas handed him a cup of water, which he drank in one gulp, his stomach heaving under his soiled garment.

He eyed the monk uneasily, then turned back to the commander. "I should talk for his sake, shouldn't I? He won't let you throw me to the wolves."

A hush fell over the room. Zosimas sat down again and appeared to be examining his sandals.

Finally, Saponas began to speak. "All right, I confess. First of all, I killed the novice Matthew." He drank another cup of water wiped his mouth on his sleeve.

Michael prompted him. "That poor boy had been lying in a church court and could no longer live with himself. As anyone present could see, his deception was making him sick. So, one of your confederated told either you, or someone spying for you. And then—"

A moan escaped Saponas. "Yes, I heard about Matthew's illness, you can be sure. Our gossip system is quicker than the Imperial Post. I knew that if Matthew told the truth, it was all over for us. So this morning I went out hunting—I said—then I reentered the city and lay in wait. I didn't know exactly when the church court would adjourn, but I was so desperate that I was willing to wait a while. I knew what route the accusers would be taking back to the monastery, and I knew of a house near the Forum of Theodosius, with a vacant second-story flat."

The Akoluthos scratched some notes on a parchment leaf, then nodded to Michael.

Michael continued the questioning. "Why did the novice Matthew slander Father Zosimas in the first place? I can guess: because someone came to the monastery and threatened him."

Saponas licked his lips. "Yes."

"Actually, I suspect they threatened his family. The youth wanted to be a monk, after all, and had almost nothing in life to lose."

Zosimas chuckled. "Oh, there's always something left to lose, even if it's only a monk's reputation."

The soldiers guffawed, but Saponas looked down at his boots. Michael cleared his throat, then posed his next question. "Will you tell us who threatened Matthew—and with what?"

Saponas pulled a face. So! Michael thought. He feels well

294

enough to play the fool again.

"I know it wasn't you, at least not directly. It was your friend Boian."

Saponas's reddened eyes widened. "You know about him too! I admit, I sent him to attend services at the monastery. He looked like a godly man—as serious and sober as a monk. He deceived everyone, I'll bet. Yes, he got in touch with Matthew."

"Again: with what did he threaten Matthew?" For the moment, Michael ignored another question that had arisen in his mind.

Saponas whispered. "Er…his parents…"

The room grew quiet, and Saponas strained to speak louder. "They have a small farm in Thrace. Or had it. Now they're tenants. They couldn't pay their taxes and were obliged to sell to a local landlord."

Michael raised an eyebrow. "A Bogomil?"

"Well…" Saponas blanched. "If Matthew didn't cooperate with Boian, the landlord would imprison his father and torture him. And evict his mother. Boian could make certain these threats were carried out."

"I repeat," said Michael. "Is this landlord a Bogomil?"

Zosimas jumped up from his seat. A blue fire burned in his eyes. "What will happen to his parents now?"

Michael had never seen Zosimas angry before. At this moment, he looked more like a soldier than a monk.

"What will happen to them?" Saponas echoed. "Nothing. Boian will have to cover his tracks now. He won't dare act… And…if I were in touch with him, I would tell him to let them be."

As though praying, Father Zosimas lifted up his hands. "Let us hope they won't be harmed!" He sank back onto the stool.

By now something else had occurred to Michael. "Saponas, when did you last see Boian?"

"Just last night. We decided that Matthew wasn't going to...work out."

"I saw Boian near the Milion Arch this noon. But where is he now?"

Saponas spread his hands. "I have no idea."

"He's not from the City, is he?"

"No, he's visiting, along with a young man called Luke."

"The grocer Peter of Serrhes claims that Luke is his cousin, as you must know," said Michael. "He and Boian appear to be staying behind the grocer's shop."

Saponas's eyes widened again. "Well, some of the time."

"Oh?" Michael was curious, but he saw Zosimas frowning in concentration and let him ask the next question.

"There's one thing I still don't understand, ah— Saponas. By the way, what's your baptismal name?"

"Nicetas."

"Nicetas—yes, I thought I'd heard it before... Why did you want to discredit me? Though I've certainly heard of you, this is the first time we've actually met. So, how have I offended you? For my part, I'm trying to forgive you, but you've caused much grief."

Saponas wiped his brow with his sleeve. "I know I owe you the truth. Um—it would be just too bad if you became Archbishop of Philippopolis. The Church couldn't have picked a better man."

Zosimas bowed his head. Michael noticed a flush cross the monk's face and wondered if anyone else did.

"Too bad for whom?" Michael asked. "The Bogomils?" Yes, too bad for them! Because Zosimas, by his unpretentious, uncalculating example, defeated all their arguments.

"Listen, Saponas," Michael continued. "I've heard you make jokes about the Old Testament, and I know what the Bogomils believe and why. You might as well admit you're one of them."

"What if I am?"

"Then we'd like to know who instigated this slander scheme. Who assigned you your part in it?" This was the question Michael had wanted to ask before.

Saponas shrugged. "Why, no one put me up to it. I was the one who recruited Boian for his task."

The Akoluthos set down his pen. "Do you expect us to believe that? Whom are you working for?" He glanced significantly at Waldemar. "We've been too polite about this business. Let's—"

Zosimas glared at the commander. "No violence!"

Michael raised a restraining hand, then addressed Saponas. "You recruited Boian—and whom else? You might as well tell us because we know already."

Saponas rolled his eyes in dismay. "Peter of Serrhes, the grocer, and his cousin. Actually, it was Luke who gave me the idea. He told me that the majority of people in the vicinity of Philippopolis want Father Zosimas as their next archbishop."

Michael raised an eyebrow. "So! It's not likely that Luke is a shepherd from the wilds near Mt. Athos. Most likely, he's from Philippopolis, the city of sin, itself."

"No doubt. Oh—it was almost perfect—" Saponas cut himself short, as though he knew his audience wouldn't appreciate his cleverness.

Michael indeed did not—and frowned. "Are Peter and Luke truly cousins?"

Saponas startled. "I never questioned the fact. But what if they aren't?"

Michael snorted. "In that case, the possibilities are intriguing."

"But not surprising," put in the Akoluthos. "Still, Saponas, you'd better tell us why you were associating with that riffraff."

"Because they're all Bogomils," said Michael.

"Is that true, Nicetas?" Zosimas inquired.

Saponas held his head high and sniffed loudly. "Yes, it is."

Michael thought his would-be pomposity came across as comic.

"But *why?*" asked Zosimas. "Why have you—?"

"Enough!" said the Akoluthos. "Only one thing concerns us about those fanatics."

Treason, Michael concluded. "I think I know how Saponas came to the Bogomil faith," said Michael. "We needn't discuss it yet. But now that we know who killed Matthew and who plotted against Father Zosimas, we can address the question that directly concerns the State: did these people also kill Bourtzes?"

298

"Yes, Saponas," said the Akoluthos. "Where were you last Monday night?"

Michael suppressed a sigh. He had cleared Zosimas, but Bourtzes's death remained a mystery. And Saponas did have a credible alibi; Michael understood that now. "You said that you were with a woman at the time of the murder, while Peter and Luke were supposedly drinking in a tavern. But you were all lying. You were all at a Bogomil prayer meeting."

A shudder racked Saponas's broad form. "You guessed."

"I presume Boian was with you."

"He's the only Perfect among us. He leads the prayers."

"How long did your meeting last?"

"From the first watch of the night until cockcrow."

Michael nodded; that made it almost impossible for them to have killed Bourtzes right after he entered the city, during the second watch of the night.

"Where did you hold your—assembly?" the Akoluthos inquired.

"That time, in an underground chamber that can be reached only through the Palace cistern."

"You will give us the names of the rest of your...faithful," said the Akoluthos. "We'll compare your story with theirs. And don't worry—we'll just terrorize them a little and let them go."

Once more, Saponas spoke. "Look—I admit to killing Matthew. I admit to plotting against Father Zosimas," he said, fixing his bloodshot eyes on Michael. "I stalked you on the west side of town last Wednesday night, and on the Palace grounds last Thursday. On Friday morning, I had my bow and positioned myself on a rooftop so I could shoot you. That failed, so I paid one of the Augusta's maids to seduce you. If I couldn't kill you, I'd disgrace you so that you couldn't testify in a church court."

So, Michael had guessed right about that, too! Still, he felt a twinge of disappointment that the girl had been bribed to pursue him.

"You didn't want me to clear Father Zosimas," he said. "I gather you didn't want me to find Bourtzes's killer either."

Saponas's stool creaked as he shifted his weight. "You're wrong. I've just confessed to committing many crimes. But I swear: I didn't kill Bourtzes, and I don't know who did."

Chapter 37

Michael threw up his hands. "If you didn't kill Bourtzes, who did? The *Kanikleios?* The Logothete of the Dromos? Tripsychos, or Metiga the Patzinak?"

Saponas managed a shrug, but regarded Michael anxiously. "I tell you—I don't know!"

Clearing his throat loudly, the Akoluthos leaned towards Saponas. "What about this Boian fellow?"

Saponas groaned, now more in weariness than pain. "He couldn't have—not in person. He was leading our prayers Monday night."

Michael inclined his head in thought. Indeed, drastic actions seemed out of character for Boian. He appeared to play the role of go-between in Saponas's plot. He had threatened Matthew, and if necessary, he would instruct the landlord to retaliate against the novice's parents. But would he actually commit murder?

The imposing, white-bearded outlander was an enigma to Michael. "Tell us more about Boian." Thus, Michael addressed Saponas. "How long have you known him?"

"Ten years, more or less."

Ten years? Perhaps that length of time was significant. "How did you meet?"

"He called on me once, when he came to the City. He travels through the west country, selling rugs."

Michael nodded. "Why did he call on you in particular?"

Saponas took a deep breath, then exhaled slowly.

"Out with it!" said the Akoluthos.

Saponas's facial muscles tensed. His eyes rested on Michael. "Boian often visited my relatives…in Dragovitsa."

"Dragovitsa, a Bogomil stronghold." Michael was not surprised, and he was glad that they were finally making progress. "Your kinsmen are Bogomils?"

"Those in Dragovitsa. But I wasn't—not then. It was Boian who introduced me to the faith." Saponas took another labored breath.

"Go on."

"I converted only five years ago. At that time, I met Peter and the others whose names I'll give you. Usually we gather in some woods, in abandoned warehouses, or in the underground cisterns."

"I see."

As Michael began to formulate his next question, Zosimas stood up, regarding Saponas with a dismayed expression. "But how could you embrace such a vile teaching. How could you believe—"

Michael raised a restraining hand. "We'll come to that. Right now, we need to know something else… Saponas, you have kin in Dragovitsa. What about in Philippopolis?"

Saponas's reddened eyes opened wide. "No."

"Surely you've journeyed that far."

"No, I haven't. I've never been to Dragovitsa either. In fact, I've never been further west than Adrianople."

Michael peered at him. "Obviously, though, you're in on the plot."

"The plot against Zosimas? I just confessed, didn't I?"

"There's more to it than Father Zosimas," said Michael.

Saponas's ragged eyebrows went up.

"Come now! First of all, the Bogomils of Philippopolis don't want Father Zosimas to go there as Archbishop. We knew that already, but you've confirmed it. You say Luke gave you the idea to slander Zosimas," said Michael.

"Yes. He came here a few weeks ago, with Boian."

"Hm!" The Akoluthos jumped up from his seat at the table. Arms crossed on his chest, he began to pace.

Saponas blanched. "Oh, I'm sure they don't want Father Zosimas there. As a Bogomil, I don't either. Luke might have given me the idea, but I'm the one who devised the defamation plot. I wasn't ordered to do it—by Luke or Boian or anyone else."

"Nonsense!" the Akoluthos roared. Then, "Waldemar, heat up that damn poker!"

Waldemar, who had been dozing against the wall, began to stretch. Zosimas moved between Saponas and the brazier.

Michael nodded in approval. "I think Saponas is telling the truth. In Father Zosimas's case, Boian was only Saponas's errand boy."

"Yes, yes!" said Saponas.

"However," Michael continued, "we have reason to believe that the Bogomils of Philippopolis are plotting secession...from the Empire. Surely you knew about *that*. Luke must have told you."

Saponas's eyes widened. "Why, no!"

"No?" Michael repeated. "He didn't? Well, perhaps the ringleaders in Philippopolis didn't tell him. If I were a traitor, I wouldn't confide in an oily little catamite."

The Akoluthos laughed.

"Still," said Michael, "it's high time we arrested the boy."

Waldemar approached the Akoluthos. "It's also time to jog Fatso's memory."

Zosimas spun around. "No, you won't!"

Waldemar gave him a stony look.

"I realize that you have a job to do," said Zosimas. "But just for a change—just this once—let's all try to behave like Christians instead of barbarian anthropophagi."

The commander's face tensed. He clenched his fists but made no move. Moments later, he flung himself into his chair. "Hell! That's enough for one night," he said, rubbing his eyes with the back of his hand. "Take the prisoner to a cell."

"I don't want to hear that he's been mistreated," said Zosimas.

A desperate light burned in Saponas's eyes. "You'll be here tomorrow?"

"If they don't throw me out." Zosimas glanced at the Akoluthos.

"Of course, they won't" Michael put in. "Until tomorrow, Saponas. We're still far from finished." Many questions in his mind clamored for an answer, but he needed time to rest, as well as time to ponder them.

§

Michael awoke at dawn, in a chamber of the ancient Daphne Palace. The frescoed walls were faded and peeling. Dust motes eddied in the pale shafts of light from the narrow windows.

Last night the room had been hastily prepared for him.

Zosimas, in the meantime had insisted on sleeping on the floor near the Varangians' jail cells...to make certain that the prisoner was not abused.

Zosimas, Michael saw, had sent him a note: he would be in the Church of the Mother of God of the Lighthouse until it was time to appear at the trial.

Michael composed a note of his own and asked a Varangian to deliver it to the Patriarch.

§

At the third hour of the day, the church court reconvened. The Patriarch scanned the chamber, then nodded in satisfaction. Surely, he noticed what Michael had already observed: Peter of Serrhes and Luke were absent.

"Today," the Patriarch began, we will continue to hear the evidence of those defending Father Zosimas. Indeed, it has been brought to our attention that Michael Taronites, who testified yesterday, has some new information."

His limbs shaking, Michael stood up. How could he be calm when Zosimas was so dear to him? "In case anyone hasn't...heard, yesterday the novice Matthew was murdered after court adjourned."

"God rest his soul," someone said. The room came alive with whispers. Garments rustled as people crossed themselves.

"Of course," said the Patriarch, "you should all pray for the poor boy's tortured soul." He turned back to Michael. "You may continue."

"Matthew took an arrow in the chest, on the way back to the monastery. But the archer was no supporter of Father Zosimas, but a man who wished to keep Matthew from telling the truth. He's since been taken into custody and has made a full confession."

"How was he questioned?" asked one of the bishops.

"Only verbally," said Michael. "Torture was not employed."

"A likely story!" said the Bishop of Cyzicus.

Zosimas sprung to his feet. "I was there," he said. "The man's confession was completely voluntary. Nobody harmed him."

"Yes," said Michael. "He—"

A rising tide of exclamations drowned out his words. Finally, the Patriarch waved the people to silence. "Go ahead, Michael."

"The man who killed Matthew is none other than the head of the Imperial household, Nicetas Saponas. He did it because Matthew had been lying in court about Father Zosimas, and he was about to break down and tell the truth. You all saw how sick he looked." He swept the chapel with a challenging gaze.

"The novice was lying in court?" asked the Bishop of Cyzicus. "Why?"

"Because his parents had been threatened," said Michael.

"Tell us how," said the Patriarch.

"They're tenants of a Bogomil landlord. Recently a Bogomil perfect called Boian came to the monastery in the guise of a humble pilgrim," Michael began and told the rest of the story.

When he had finished, one of the bishops furrowed his brow. "You say that Saponas directed the whole slander

306

campaign, and that Peter and Luke willingly played their parts? Where are they now?"

"I wonder." Michael looked behind him. Others also searched in vain for the grocer and the youth.

"So," began the Patriarch. "I think we can dismiss the charges brought by the first two plaintiffs as completely false."

A shout of approval went up. "Aye!"

But the Patriarch's face darkened. "However, we're not entirely finished."

Michael nodded. What *were* they going to do about Father Jonas?

Right at that moment, Jonas staggered to his feet. "Your Holiness," he began, wiping a strand of sweat-soaked hair from his chalky brow. "I wish to withdraw my accusation. That night I didn't see what I thought I saw. I was deceived by the devil, and later I was influenced by the false gossip circulating in the monastery."

"Now, Father," put in the Bishop of Cyzicus, "you can't just make an accusation and then withdraw it on a mere whim. When you brought your testimony before the court, you agreed to accept the defendant's canonical penalty if he were found innocent."

Jonas buried his face in his hands and wept. "Oh, you can defrock me if you like. Do with me what you will. Just give me leave to retire to the wilderness—where I can live in solitude and repent of my poor judgment and my sins."

What an actor! Michael thought. He ought to play Oedipus Rex.

The Patriarch nodded. The distended vein on his brow

had all but vanished. "Yes, we will see to it that you are confined to a place of repentance. But now I propose that we drop all charges against Father Zosimas of the Studion as ill-founded and deliberately slanderous."

§

Michael escorted a weak, bemused Father Zosimas out of the chapel, ahead of the rest of the assembly. A servant seated them in a small reception room and promptly brought the monk a cup of water.

Michael patted Zosimas on the shoulder. "It's over—thank God—and you've been cleared."

Zosimas merely smiled.

"Now the whole world will know that the charges against you were false," said Michael. "I regret only that Father Jonas did not confess his offense against your person."

Zosimas waved dismissively. "I told you—I'm sure it was only a momentary temptation. It's good that he wants to repent. If he confesses his sin to a priest, it will be sufficient."

Michael scowled. "But he must have borne a grudge against you. Why else would he accuse you?"

"Well—"

"Do you think he'll be deposed?" asked Michael.

"Oh, I doubt it. He'll be suspended for a time—even years—but that may be all."

Michael rose from his seat and paced the floor. "Some of us aren't let off so easily. We go on paying for our follies."

"You mean...Barbara."

"Yes. So far Lady Olympia has made no attempt to

contact me."

"Oh." Zosimas set down his cup and stared into the distance. "God willing, she'll repent of her obstinacy—or whatever—if she's everything she seems to be."

"Oh, she is," said Michael, resting his bearded chin on his chest. "But I do understand her. If I were in her position, I would be disgusted. Whatever happens between us, I would prefer that she not think of me as a swine."

"You're not a swine," said Zosimas, "but only human, like the rest of us. Just as she is. Still, why don't you try—"

The rest of his thought remained unspoken. They heard a murmur outside, then the shuffle of sandaled feet.

Michael rose as the white-bearded Abbot of the Studion, several monks, and the Abbess Anastasia came in. Zosimas also stood and exchanged the kiss of peace with his sister and the Abbot.

"Thank God you've been cleared!" said the nun. Then, with a smiling glance at Michael, she added, "And thank you for defending my little brother."

Michael bowed. "I did what I could."

"Well!" the Abbot addressed Zosimas. "Now you might be leaving us."

Zosimas startled. "Why would I?"

"What if they make you Archbishop of Philippopolis?"

Zosimas blinked and smiled a faint, beautiful smile. "That remains to be seen."

Chapter 38

That afternoon, Olympia made a sick call at the Great Palace. The Emperor's mistress had sent word to the Court physician's office that she was ill. Acropolites, who had been nursing the Emperor, through another siege of gout, felt too weary to deal with the whims of the pampered Augusta and dispatched his student in his stead.

The Alan lady languished under a blanket of marten fur, her straight blond hair spread out on a silk-covered pillow. Olympia placed a hand on her forehead and found it hot and dry. The Augusta was truly ill, then.

There were times, though, when indigestion—actually gluttony—or her monthly courses subjected her to untold agonies. Olympia could sympathize with the latter complaint.

Today, however, she needed to seek the cause of the Augusta's malady. First, she took the lady's pulse in her wrist, then pulled back the coverlet and sounded her chest; it was clear. Last of all, she prodded the Augusta's abdomen, but found no lump or swelling there.

"Still, I ache," said the Augusta.

"It will pass." Olympia took her apothecary box from her bag, emptied a small vial of willow juice into a pitcher of water, and gave the patient a cup. "Stay in bed and drink this as you need it. We'll be back to see you in a day or so."

Olympia feared that this attempt at healing was not one of her more inspired and quit the Augusta's apartments in haste. She wished only to return to the physician's office and do some work. She had nothing else to look forward to.

On her way to the Brazen Gates, she passed through the courtyard of the Sigma. Several officials stood by the wine-flowing fountain, talking in low voices.

Today she'd seen many such groups on the Palace grounds. Once or twice, she'd overheard someone say that the Varangians had made an important arrest: important in reference to what?

But on her way here, out in the Augusteum, she had heard whisperings of a different kind: all charges against Father Zosimas were being dropped.

She was certain that Michael had played some part in this. What had he discovered? If she ever found out, it would be from others. How could she face him again, after her outburst? And how could he face *her*? What man could dismiss such an insult—indeed, any insult?

Still, everything was not permitted to men simply because they were men. So, she had always believed and always would. But she had not been fair to Michael.

And she had not been fair to herself when she dismissed her feeling for him as lust. Unlike the blaze of lust, her affection had not consumed itself. Nor would it ever, despite his shortcomings—despite hers, which she now saw clearly. And regardless of whatever happened between them—or did not happen—her feeling was a white, cleansing fire stronger than death, a fire that would never burn out.

She had just entered a covered walkway, when a twig snapped somewhere outside it. She started, and the long strap of her bag slipped down her arm. Who was following her?

She looked through the columns of the passageway and saw no one. Out on the fading lawn, the branches of a yew tree waved in the still air.

"Yes?" she called.

No answer came.

Olympia was not frightened but annoyed. Who was playing childish games with her? She threw the strap of her bag over her shoulder and set off again, watching the tree out of the corner of her eye.

A moment later, a woman's voice hailed her. "Lady?"

She turned, and the branches shifted again. A slender young woman, wrapped in a plain cloak fastened with a pewter brooch, emerged from behind the yew. "Lady?" She bowed with the studied formality of a servant, then hurried towards Olympia.

"You're a doctor, aren't you?"

"Almost. I'm a student," said Olympia.

"And you're name's Macrembolitissa?"

"It is." *Just what did this girl want?*

"Good! Well, my friend has some female trouble. Maybe you can help her." She looked towards a stand of evergreen trees and waved. "It's all right!"

Olympia slumped her shoulders. "I supposed I can give her some advice." *For all that I know about women's problems!*

An olive-skinned, petite figure emerged from the trees. Olympia felt a twinge of inner pain, for she recognized her at once.

"I'll be going now," said the first girl, and vanished.

Before Olympia could speak, the small woman was

beside her on the walkway. Her saffron-colored headscarf fell back, revealing thick dark hair plaited around her head.

"Lady Olympia, my name is Barbara. We haven't exactly met, but I think we have—ah—a mutual friend." She looked quickly away and rearranged her kerchief.

"I presume you mean Michael Taronites." Olympia managed a sad smile. Somehow the girl soothed her anguish. She was friendly, but neither haughty or forward.

"Are you his betrothed?"

Olympia flinched. What a charitable question—not like what she'd asked Michael: "Is that your mistress?"

"No, he's not. We just work together sometimes."

"Are your parents against it?" Barbara inquired. But as soon as the words were out, she covered her mouth with her hand.

"Well, yes. Or at least my father is. He wants me to marry a self-important fool, with money. He—"

She broke off, and flushed. What had possessed her to discuss her personal affairs with a stranger, and one considered beneath her station? But somehow it felt right; somehow it eased her heart.

"I would guess that you love him—I mean—Lord Michael. But I think that the two of you have...had words because of me."

Olympia startled. "How do you know?"

"I saw you together. On Monday, the first day of Father Zosimas's trial."

"Yes. That's when I saw you."

"I swear—it was a chance meeting. I joined the crowds because I'd heard about Father Zosimas and felt sorry for him. I hadn't seen Mi—er—Lord Taronites for years, but I heard he was going to testify. When I happened to see him, I wanted to give him my greetings."

"I—is that so?" Olympia's head swam, and she sank onto the stone bench to one side of the walkway.

"May I..." Barbara wrung her hands. When Olympia nodded, she sat down a good two feet away. "It's true," she said. "There's nothing between us now. I swear it."

Olympia took a deep breath, trying to control her inner turmoil. "You don't have to swear. I believe you."

"What did he tell you, Lady?"

"About you? Only that he'd...known you years ago. He blamed everything on his own folly, not on you. You were sinned against, not sinning, he said. He also claimed that the incident led to his father's arrest. I regret that at first I didn't believe him."

Barbara winced. "I tricked him—as part of Michael the Caulker's scheme. He—" Quickly she averted her gaze. Just as quickly, Olympia placed a hand on his shoulder. "Go on."

Barbara backed away, looking Olympia straight in the eye. "Lord Taronites wasn't to blame. He thought he loved me—poor boy that he was. And he was the only man in the Palace that treated me as a person, instead of just dirt."

Olympia signed. "I believe you." She had misjudged Michael, and the woman's words confirmed Olympia's first understanding of him. While some men, like the Emperor, emulated the manners of the coarse and the vulgar, Michael treated the humble and the simple as his equals—and raised them to his level. "Yes, he's fair-minded, not haughty or snobbish. It's only those who intentionally do evil, those who harm others, that he can't abide."

Barbara blinked; was she holding back tears? "I repaid him with treachery. I...kept him from meeting his father, and the poor man had no alibi for the time they said he—"

"But you were forced to."

"Still, it was wicked. I take the blame."

Olympia clasped the woman's slender hand. "Michael also wishes to take the whole blame. But in my opinion, both of you are being entirely too noble. We all make mistakes—all of us."

Barbara lowered her eyes momentarily, then faced Olympia again. "You still love him—I can tell! Just don't let him go. You won't find a better man."

"I thank you for your...help. No one could find a better, more honest woman than you." Olympia released her grasp, and Barbara rose to go.

"Thank you for listening to me, Lady. Now I've got to get back to my little boy." Barbara slipped out between two columns and padded over the dry grass, disappearing into a clump of cypress trees.

When Olympia returned to the office, she found Acropolites waiting for her. "Someone left a message especially for you."

Olympia hung up her cloak, but her curiosity drew her back to the doctor. "Who?"

"He looked like someone's servant, but I didn't recognize him. Here!" He handed her a small scroll.

She sat down at the table and cut the seal with a penknife, then unrolled the letter. A lamp supplemented the fading daylight.

As she read the salutation, her fingers dug into the parchment leaf; it was from Bourtzes's widow.

Her request appeared simple. "Lately I have been suffering from sleeplessness, and today I am quite unwell. Please come as soon as possible, with more of your teacher's potion."

"Well!" She dropped the note into her bag.

Chapter 39

Afternoon found Michael back at the Palace, in the Varangians' interrogation room. Once again, Saponas occupied a low stool, and once again, Zosimas was present—with reluctant official permission.

The Akoluthos tapped his pen on the desk top. "Well, Saponas, we don't think much of your friends. The militia can't find Boian, and Peter and Luke have also vanished."

"Oh?" Michael asked. But somehow, he was not surprised.

Saponas's jaw dropped. "I know nothing about it."

The Akoluthos grimaced. "I'll bet." He turned to Michael. "Last night, after you left, I took some men to arrest the grocer and his cousin. They were gone."

"What about Peter's wife?"

"Oh, she was there all right. We woke her up. She said Peter came home yesterday noon."

"After the trial," Michael added. He knew that the militia had gone there after Matthew's death.

"The woman says that after the militia left, Peter and Luke put her in charge of the shop. They went out and never came back."

"Did Boian come by and warn them to get out of town?"

"I don't know," said the Akoluthos. "Nor does Peter's wife. Boian could have entered their living quarters while she was out in the shop. But she hasn't seen him in either place since last Friday."

"When I first saw him," said Michael. "But we know that

he was in town as late as yesterday noon."

"I doubt he is now," said the Akoluthos. "No one was hiding on the grocer's premises, and most of Peter and Luke's belongings were gone. Earlier the woman hadn't noticed that they'd cleaned out their storage chests."

"So, they must have left the City last night before the gates closed," said Michael. "And by the way, does this poor woman have a name?"

The Akoluthos rubbed his blond beard and thought for a moment. "Irene. And we let her go free. She must be innocent."

"I believe so," said Michael. "When I spoke to her, she seemed completely ignorant of their activities. And I would guess that Peter is a miser and a wife-beater. I doubt she misses him."

"And he doesn't miss her!" Waldemar added with a chuckle. "Luke is Peter's wife." The other Varangians guffawed.

Father Zosimas, who was sitting on a stool, looked down at his sandals. "Er—that's possible, of course."

"So! Saponas," Michael began, "Were they actually related? Do you know?"

Once more, Saponas shrugged. "I really don't know. Peter did introduce the boy as his cousin, but he came to the City with Boian. Certainly, the three of them are brother Bogomils, but Peter might have claimed the boy as his cousin so that the Eparch's office would let him stay here."

"True," said Michael. Unlike Boian, who at least posed as a rug merchant, he had no legitimate business here. But why did he come here in the first place? To make his fortune?

The Akoluthos grunted. "He found a protector."

"But did he also have a political motive? We know of one plot he was involved in."

"We may never know," said the Akoluthos. "It seems they've slipped our snares. But we'll notify the provincial authorities. If they catch the scum—"

"If not, the pair of them won't come back," Michael concluded. "They've been identified as Bogomils, and they lied in an ecclesiastical court. And Boian is a known Bogomil."

Saponas's eyes widened, as if something obscure had suddenly become clear to him. "You know, I think that from the time we conceived the plot against Father Zosimas, they always planned to escape together. They never said anything, but I always felt that there was something unspoken between them."

"Well!" Michael tensed, because the memory of the trial still rankled. "Of course, you didn't expect to be implicated. You were only the hidden hand."

Saponas bowed his head. "Yes."

Now the Akoluthos broke in. "Taronites, you've omitted something. Did they kill Bourtzes?"

"No."

"They couldn't have," put in Saponas. "As I said, we were all together that night."

The Akoluthos scrawled a note and set down his pen. "We did learn something new about your Boian."

Saponas regarded him with curiosity.

"The Eparch's office knows a man answering to Boian's

description. He's called Svetoslav of Chomatini, and he comes to the City every year to sell Peloponnesian carpets. He claims residence in the Peloponnese, not in Chomatini, his supposed place of origin."

Saponas threw up his hands. "I've never heard that name, though I knew he sold rugs."

"He's most probably a Bulgar by birth and known by that name back home. Or it could be a false name. Now I'll wager that he'll find a new name, as well as a new business."

The Akoluthos nodded. "He has plenty to answer for, but he and his friends couldn't have killed Bourtzes... Fatso here is telling the truth." He glared in Saponas's direction, shaking his fist.

A shiver of fear crossed Saponas's broad face. "I swear. It's as I told you!"

"Enough!" Michael shot a reproving glance at the commander, then turned back to Saponas. "We have no reason to doubt what you've told us. But you may know more than you're saying—or more than you think you know. So, let's concentrate on our other suspects."

Saponas scratched his shaggy beard. "What do you mean?"

"Think of the two courtiers, Blachernites and Syropoulos. And of Tripsychos, the Postal agent. And the Patzinak lord. Are any of them Bogomils?"

"None of them ever came to our prayer meetings," replied Saponas, "so I wouldn't know. Anyway, aren't the Patzinaks heathens? At least..."

"At least what?" demanded Michael.

"At least the ones I know."

"And who are *they*?" Michael recalled now that at the Emperor's reception, Saponas had joked about drinking *koumis* with some Patzinaks.

"Last spring, when I stayed at an inn on the Adrianople road, I made the acquaintance of that Uzun fellow and some of his friends. At the time I didn't know he was related to Metiga."

"And what did you do?"

"We drank a skin of *koumis*. It was awful. I nearly puked."

Michael nodded. Saponas had remarked that the stuff tasted like mare's piss, not mare's milk.

The Akoluthos rapped the table. "We don't care what slops those savages drink. Are they Bogomils?"

Saponas groaned. "I said they're heathens."

A dense, weary feeling washed over Michael. He shook his head to dispel it. He could not rid himself of the thought that the Bogomil heresy had some connection with Bourtzes's death, but it appeared less and less likely. He would have to backtrack in his questioning.

"Saponas, I'll repeat a question I asked you last night. Did Luke ever discuss secession from the Empire?"

"No!"

The Akoluthos slammed the table. "Is that true?"

"I swear!"

"All right," said Michael. "Now, what were you doing on the Adrianople Road?"

"I have relatives in Adrianople. I went to visit them. Don't worry—they're not Bogomils but as pious as you like."

Michael slumped his shoulders; he was making no progress. Then, "What about Leo Syropoulos? Did you know that his ancestors were Paulicians?"

Saponas's eyes widened. "No!"

"They weren't Syrians, but Armenians from Argaoun, a Paulician settlement. Syropoulos does his best to conceal the fact, which makes me wonder about him. You see, his origins aren't really a source of shame; his ancestors abandoned their heresy and fought for the Empire."

"He's certainly hidden it well," said Saponas. "But..."

"But what?" Michael demanded. "He's a pederast? And who's that boy, anyway?"

"I don't know about his private life. I presume that boy is a servant."

The Akoluthos chuckled. "Syropoulos claims that he's an old family retainer, or at least the son of his chief horse groom."

Michael turned to the Varangian. "So you know more about him than Saponas."

"Well," Saponas continued, "all I can say about Syropoulos is that he's a haughty one. He needs a swift kick in the...well, never mind." He cast a shamefaced glance at Father Zosimas.

Zosimas smiled faintly, and addressed the prisoner. "Do you have any reason to believe that Syropoulos is himself a Paulician?"

Saponas replied with a shrug.

Michael frowned. "Of course, if I were any such thing, I'd conceal it."

"Well—" Saponas stretched, and leaned back in his

chair.

"Nicetas," put in Zosimas, "you never told us why you joined the Bogomil sect."

"There's not much to tell."

"Isn't there, where such a fateful decision is concerned?"

"Go on," said Michael.

The Akoluthos made a derisive snort.

"As I said, I was still running the soapworks when I met Boian—about ten years ago. From time to time we'd talk, but it was only after I was called to the Palace that I converted."

The Akoluthos leaned forward, planting his elbows on the table. "What do you do at your Bogomil services?"

"We pray and read the New Testament."

"What prayers do you say?" asked Zosimas.

"Mostly 'Our Father.'"

"Giving the words your own allegorical interpretation," the monk concluded.

The Akoluthos broke in again. "Wait—don't the Bogomils...wicked orgies?" He glanced uneasily at Zosimas.

"Aren't they all buggers?" put in Waldemar.

Zosimas cleared his throat. "We're not here to trade nasty stories."

"Oh, that!" For a moment Saponas looked about to tell a lewd joke, but then put on a serious expression. "I have never encountered any such things. Perhaps they occur in private."

"This does not concern us," said the monk. "We were discussing Bogomil practice and doctrines."

"What does that nonsense have to do with this case?" The Akoluthos demanded.

Zosimsa raised a restraining hand. "I want to learn how he came to believe in Bogomil teachings."

Saponas looked away. "It's hard to explain."

Michael didn't doubt his words. Though Saponas was certainly clever and cunning, serious thought was not a habit with him. Still, Michael suspected that Saponas, beneath his comic mask, was a man of some feeling. "Just try your best."

"Well..." Saponas rolled his eyes, then regarded Zosimas in earnest. "I suppose I grew up just like everything else. I thought that God ruled the world, assisted by his Vice-Regent, the Emperor. But mind you, I didn't dwell much on that—or anything else. I was carefree and took things as they came."

That Michael believed.

"Little by little I realized that things weren't what they ought to be. Out in the countryside, the rich preyed upon the poor, while here in the Capital, everyone had his fun. The Empress Zoe took lovers and poisoned her first husband, and then, before we knew it, we were plagued with monsters—namely, John the Orphanotrophus and his nephew, Michael the Caulker. They mutilated, tortured, and killed many innocent people. Where was the justice in that?"

"There was none whatsoever," Zosimas replied, "as you believed yourself. You led an army of soapmakers against the Caulker, didn't you?"

Michael wondered what Zosimas was leading up to.

324

"I did," replied Saponas. "That fiend didn't deserve to rule."

"Of course not," said Michael. "No one here will argue with that."

"But it wasn't just what was happening out in the world that was wrong. It was what took place in my own house."

Zosimas inclined his head to one side and awaited Saponas's next words.

"You may recall that ten years ago, a visitation of smallpox came upon the City…" He broke off and lowered his eyes.

Yes, Michael recalled that Saponas's son had mentioned the epidemic. And now he saw that Saponas wept. "I know," he said. "You lost your wife and all but one of your children."

Saponas breathed deeply, as though glad he didn't have to say the words himself, then wiped his eyes on his sleeve. "How do you—"

"I talked with your son."

Saponas looked up. "Oh. But the worst was—"

"You didn't catch it at all, and wished that you'd been afflicted in their stead."

Saponas bowed his head in acknowledgment. Everyone kept silent; Michael could hear the lamps sputter. The Akoluthos shifted his weight, and a sad, knowing look crossed Zosimas's face.

Finally, Saponas spoke. "Why? They'd done no evil."

Zosimas stood up. "So, you came to believe that while a good God rules the spiritual world, an evil god rules the material."

Saponas's voice was hoarse. "An evil god, or the devil. Satanel!"

Zosimas flinched at the dread Bogomil term and quickly crossed himself. "The devil is not God's equal," he said, "but only a creature." The Varangians stirred uneasily, as though the devil were indeed in the room with them.

Michael could follow Saponas's argument. He was actually beginning to pity the man. But now he spoke with no little rancor. "Father Zosimas never did anyone any harm either, but that didn't stop evil tongues from attacking him. In both your case and his, we know the agent of evil; it certainly wasn't God—or any god."

Zosimas placed a hand on Michael's shoulder. "Leave me out of this. I never did the things they accused me of, but I have many sins. That's why God allowed this misfortune to befall me."

The Akoluthos struck the table with his fist. "Enough, Father! Let's not hear your confession as well."

Michael agreed. Who in the present company could follow the monk's train of thought? Who could comprehend what he considered to be his sins?

"All I meant," Michael said, "was that God is not the author of evil. Wicked people caused Father Zosimas's difficulties, and a hideous illness caused Saponas's."

"Such things occur because the universe is at war with itself," said Zosimas. "Though it was created by a good God, man fell and dragged down the rest of creation with him."

Saponas blinked. Otherwise he did not react. "Somehow I took my misfortunes to heart."

"Who wouldn't have?" asked Zosimas.

"I lost all joy in life, but I went on living. I spent more time with Boian. Though I'd previously ignored his preaching, I now heeded it with one ear. I lived that way for a few years."

"Then the Emperor, Michael IV died, and Michael the Caulker, his nephew, seized the throne and began to wreak havoc. When the people learned that he'd imprisoned the Empress Zoe, his adopted mother, they rose up against him. Well, Zoe was an old whore—"

"Stop!" warned the Akoluthos. "You're defaming the Imperial Majesty." Yet he didn't protest very strenuously.

Michael, on the other hand, felt that he should mention the Empress's good points. "She was always kind to my father and me, as well as to many others."

"Ah—excuse me," put in Saponas. "I admit—whatever she was, she was still a better person than the Caulker. And she was from a good family—the ruling family. So, I wanted to help her. So, I gathered my fellow soapmakers, inflamed them against the tyrant, and marched them to the Palace armed with vat stirrers, hunting bows, sticks and stones, and whatever knives they could find in their kitchens."

"And thus, you became a hero," said Michael.

"Yes. The Empress Zoe awarded me with money. After she married Monomachus, and he ascended the throne, he promoted me to the Senate and made me the head of his household. I think he liked me from the start because I was a good mimic, actor, and jester. The filthier my jokes were, the funnier he thought them."

Zosimas rested his brow in his hands.

"Well, you see," continued Saponas, "I knew the Vice-

Regent of God for a drunkard and a skirt-chaser. I wasn't the only fool in the Palace."

The Akoluthos sprung to his feet. "Watch your tongue if you want to keep it! That's *lèse-majesté* again!"

Saponas's lip trembled only slightly. "It was then that I joined the Bogomils. Their beliefs made more and more sense to me. God created only the invisible world, while the visible world—and man—were created by the devil. If there's any hope for us wretches, it lies in escaping the material. Let the small spark of the spirit—of light—if there be any imprisoned in our vile carcasses, return to its source!"

Satisfied that he'd hear no more treason, the Akoluthos sat down. He concealed a yawn behind his hand.

"Nicetas!" said Zosimas. "Know that your faith is without hope. It's a faith of constant strife between darkness and light."

Could anyone live without hope? Michael wondered. If one did not believe that ultimately God would defeat the devil, that light would overcome darkness, then all one's efforts were in vain.

Hope was indispensable in one's own life as well. If Michael did not believe he could be reconciled with Olympia, then surely he'd lost her forever. Hope was also necessary in temporal affairs: if one did not believe in the possibility of justice despite all indications to the contrary, how could one fight for it?

And if Michael did not believe he could find Bourtzes's murderer—

"Taronites!" demanded the Akoluthos. "Are you

awake?"

"Ah—yes."

"I was just asking the prisoner what kind of hell he raised in the Palace."

Saponas took a sip of water. "My new religion didn't affect my role there at all; as you know, Bogomils are encouraged to deceive the servants of the devil by whatever means. So, in addition to managing the Imperial household, I also pleased His Majesty by devising the most vulgar jokes and entertainments imaginable. At the same time, I laughed behind his back—behind everyone's back. People's behavior only confirmed my beliefs."

Zosimas sighed. "If only our rulers understood that whether they're good or bad, we look to them as examples. And when they scandalize us—"

Again, the Akoluthos slammed his fist on the table. "We'll have none of that talk! We're sworn to protect the Emperor."

Michael faced him. "Do you really think that this monk would lift a finger against the consecrated person of the Autocrator?"

The Varangian's expression relaxed, but he didn't reply. Then the clock out in the Augusteum rang out the ninth hour, and he swore under his breath. "This has gone on long enough. Dismissed!"

Two Varangians took hold of Sapons and dragged him to his feet. For an instant, his florid face went pale. "Father! Will you visit me in my cell?"

"I will."

Michael wondered why Saponas wanted the monk near

him. To protect him from torture? To make a favorable impression on his captors? Or was there another reason?

In any case, Michael now understood why Zosimas had asked the former soapmaker about his attack on the Palace. "Saponas!" he called out. "I don't think you ever gave up hope—for justice or for some sort of good. Why did you march against the Caulker?"

"I don't know why. And here's a question for you people: why did an all-good God create such an evil world. *That* you've never been able to answer."

"Nicetas, wait—" said Zosimas, but the guards marched Saponas past him, out of the room.

When the door slammed behind him, Michael threw up his hands. "Now what?"

"Now you go out and find Bourtzes's killer," said the Akoluthos.

As if it were that simple!

"Taronites, you're the one who told me that this crime was mixed up with the plot against the monk. Now it seems it's not."

"So I believed." Michael began to laugh recklessly; his position was sublimely absurd. He stopped only when someone rapped on the door.

"Come in," said the Akoluthos.

The door swung open, admitting the white-haired Logothete of the Dromos. He looked around warily. "Taronites…"

"Your Excellency…" Despite his reservations, Michael bowed deeply. But once again, the Logothete showed no respect to Father Zosimas. And what was he doing here, anyway? Trying to discover what they'd learned? Alas, if he were truly guilty of Bourtzes's death, he'd be reassured.

But the Logothete's face was unreadable. "I wanted to let you know that Tripsychos came in this afternoon. I advised him not to leave the Palace until you'd spoken with him."

"Thank you, sir. I'll find him."

Now the Akoluthos broke in. "So you'll be on your way, Taronites. And enough of this Bogomil shit." He glanced at Father Zosimas. "Oh—sorry. We'll see that you get back to the monastery."

A whirlwind of suspicions assailed Michael as he walked from the Varangians' headquarters back to the Post. Had the Logothete killed Bourtzes, and was he trying to divert suspicion from himself?

But was he truly guilty of Bourtzes's death? Why would he have killed the man? Michael found it hard to believe that the man was a Bogomil; he had a common-sense aversion to any sort of quackery or sects. Motive aside, however, he was one of the three men who knew of Bourtzes's mission, and he had a weak alibi for the time of the agent's death.

On the other hand, what of Syropoulos's loud denials of anything to do with the Paulician heretics—and what of his pretty-boy servant?

And what of the silent, brooding man Michael was about to see?

By now Michael had reached the Post. A night guard, who had just come on duty, admitted him with a nod. In the corridor, hanging lamps cast a yellow glow on the unadorned walls, but dark doorways yawned on either side.

As he ascended to the second floor, his footsteps reverberated loudly against the walls of the stairwell.

A soft light shone under the door he sought, at the far end of the hall.

Michael knocked briskly on the heavy oak planks. "It's Taronites."

"Come in."

Michael paused on the threshold of the tiny room. Tripsychos was slumped in his desk chair, his head bowed. A pungent herbal scent hung in the air.

He looked up, nodding towards an extra chair. His dark, curly hair was damp around his temples. "Please, sit down," he said. "Would you like some refreshment?"

"No thank you." *Because I don't know what you'll put in it.*

"I'm drinking watered wine with honey." Tripsychos indicated a pewter cup on his desk, next to some parchments. "It makes my medicine more pleasant."

"I see." Michael stole a curious glance at his host—or prey. The man's skin had a yellowish cast, noticeable even in the dim lamplight. He moved slowly, as a man in pain. But was his illness the sole source of his discomfort?

"How's your wound? Any better?"

Tripsychos's shrug was barely noticeable. "Perhaps. I don't have the rot, but the fever won't go away."

"I hope it does soon." What else could Michael say?

"Well, I'm growing weary." Tripsychos leaned back in his chair and stretched his long legs in front of him. "No doubt I should stay in bed, but I can't."

Michael felt his spirits sinking; the other man's pain

affected him. "I'm sorry. I won't keep you long, but I think you know why I've come."

Tripsychos looked up. "Yes."

"Originally, I wanted to know your whereabouts yesterday noon—I was told that you were at home—but that's no longer relevant. Saponas has confessed to killing the novice Matthew—murdered yesterday at noon—and to conspiring against Father Zosimas."

"Saponas?" Tripsychos's somber, liquid eyes, seemed unusually large. "Why?"

Michael winced. "Do you really not know?"

"No." His eyes narrowed.

"Oh." Michael's shoulders slumped. "By the way, Saponas did not kill Bourtzes, and whoever did is still at large."

Tripsychos sat up. "In other words, I'm still under suspicion."

"Yes—as a formality." Michael would have preferred not to torture the man with questions, but he knew he must. "And we're still interested in your whereabouts last Monday night."

"As I said, I went to St. John's Hospital to have my dressing changed. It was during the second watch of the night, and by the third, I was home."

Michael eyed him significantly. "That's what's in our records. And you live close by the hospital, in the Psamathia quarter." *Close enough, so that with careful timing, you could have ridden hard over the fields lying between it and the beech grove...and back again.*

"My servants saw me leave that night. They were asleep

when I came home."

"How many servants do you have?"

"Two—an older couple."

"Much like mine, then." He knew from reading the Varangians' report that that like him, Tripsychos lived in a rather small house. Also, like Michael, Tripsychos was a man of modest means. "Aside from them, you live alone?"

A shadow crossed his face. "You know that."

"So, we have only your word."

"Please!"

"I know you're a widower," said Michael. "However, before you were married, you paid court to the woman who later became Bourtzes's wife. You loved her."

Tripsychos sprang up. The cords in his neck tensed. "That was a childish infatuation."

Michael also jumped to his feet, ready to ward of any blows.

"She means nothing to me now," Tripsychos said. "I consider myself better off as I am."

"Is that so? Why, then, did you engage in that famous fist-fight with Bourtzes in the halls of the Post?"

Tripsychos slowly exhaled. "That was years ago! But at the time, I was angry because he got everything first— everything! Assignments, wives, glory..."

And death.

"I know it was foolish of me to hit him then, but once I did, he had to defend himself."

"Of course."

"So, I paid him back in kind, and then there was no stopping it. When I think of the curses we used—it was madness."

"Ahem—yes."

"As I said, I know I'm better off as I am."

But Michael understood that he had opened a wound. And this man of few words had been a man of choleric temperament. Was he still? Had he changed at all?

"In that case," said Michael, "have you ever thought of entering a monastery?"

"Sometimes."

Michael hadn't expected that. But, still, even though he hated the role he played, he proceeded. "However, sometimes one wonders, or one doubts. Isn't that so? Why did an all-good God create such a wicked world, and why does He allow so much evil to take place?" He would see if he were dealing with another Bogomil.

Tripsychos snorted disdainfully and turned away. "Really! A child knows better than that. The world was created good in the beginning. And as for the evils of this life—whether we live or die, we belong to God."

Michael blinked. He hadn't expected this either. Could it possibly be a sham?

Finally, he recovered himself enough to speak. "Perhaps you should speak with Saponas, then. He has problems of belief."

Tripsychos stared back at him.

"Saponas is a Bogomil," said Michael, studying the look of frank surprise that crossed Tripsychos's face.

Chapter 40

A t the end of the working day, Olympia felt obliged to keep the peace with her father. But, after supper, she announced that she had to deliver some medicines for Acropolites and, with her two eunuchs, set off for Bourtzes's house in the carriage. She did not foresee that she would be gone long, and she assumed that while she was occupied, they could visit with the widow's household servants.

The widow Marina awaited her in the reception room, her slender hands clutching the back of a carved teakwood chair. "Thank God you've come!"

"Lady," began Olympia, "I received your message, and I brought you some sleeping potion." Fingering the strap of her bag, Olympia studied Marina's sallow skin, and the black hollows beneath her eyes. But there was something else in the widow's face, something extraordinary.

"Ah—can you come upstairs?"

"Of course," said Olympia. Her stomach clenched. Something was amiss here: the lady was incoherent, perhaps even distracted. She mustn't be allowed to neglect or harm herself.

Marina, her black gown swirling around her, led Olympia up the stone staircase, stopping only at the third floor. Then, looking back to make certain Olympia was still there, she hurried down a lamplit corridor, pausing at a door near the end.

Why here?

They entered, and Olympia surveyed the room quickly:

a vanity table, a bed with a silk coverlet, a chair or two, benches piled high with cushions, a light-colored Persian rug—a lady's room. Marina's.

"Please sit down," the widow said.

"Thank you." Olympia pushed some pillows aside and sat down on a bench, her bag beside her. "You sit down too. Those are doctor's orders."

Marina picked up her vanity chair and sat down across from Olympia.

"I fear you're ill," said Olympia, "and I think you should call your own physician. I'm still a student. Though I can give general advice, I can practice only under the direction of my teacher."

"I understand. But doesn't he want you to be here?" Marina buried her face in a handkerchief.

Olympia stood up, and embraced Marian. "I know you weep. I know no words can take the pain away. But I want to help."

Marina mumbled against Olympia's shoulder. "You said you would."

"I did." Olympia led Marina to the bench and sat down beside her. What was wrong?

"The medicine..." Marina began, dabbing at her eyes with the handkerchief.

"The medicine." As Olympia repeated the words, she observed Marina. "I find it hard to believe that you have trouble sleeping."

"I do."

Olympia gasped. Only now did she realize what was extraordinary about Marina's appearance. Her eyes were bloodshot from weeping—yes. But her pupils were tiny. "I don't think you need any more of the poppy," Olympia said, "not for a good while. You used what I gave you—and obtained more, no doubt, from your own physician."

Marina, opened her mouth, but no sound came.

Olympia nodded, confirming the situation to herself, then addressed the widow. She rose. "Tell me, is your maid available?"

"Yes." She picked up a handbell from the table, went to the door, and rang it. "Christina?"

Moments later, a slender, blonde girl in her late teens appeared.

"Mistress?"

Olympia broke in. "Christina—Please! Go to the kitchen and have them heat some water to boiling. Bring us a pitcher-full, some cups, spoons, and a strainer."

"Yes, ma'am."

Olympia closed the door behind her, then turned to Marina, seizing her by the wrists. "You're poisoning yourself. Too much can stop your breathing. Or do you seek…oblivion?"

Struggling against Olympia's grip, Marina looked away.

"No oblivion, no sleep lasts forever," Olympia said. "Not even death. In the end, we're left with what we know."

Sobbing deeply, Marina flung herself on Olympia's shoulder.

"You can lighten your burden. If you tell someone what grieves you…"

Marina pulled away. "I need someone I can trust."

"Trust?"

"Someone who won't tell a soul."

For a moment, Olympia hesitated. "Did you want to tell me? Is that why you wanted me to come?"

Marina turned away.

"But you couldn't quite summon up the courage."

Marina stuffed her handkerchief into her sleeve and faced Olympia again. "Do you swear— Doctors can keep secrets," she said, taking Marina's hands again. "They hold to the oath of the ancient teacher Hippocrates: 'Whatever I see or hear, professionally or privately, which ought not to be divulged, I will keep secret and tell no one.' So, you see, your confidences are as safe with me as with a priest, under the seal of confession."

Olympia's grip slackened. Marina collapsed against her and began to weep anew. Olympia tried to keep her mounting curiosity at bay; like a midwife attending a difficult birth, she could only wait. Until the womb had fully opened and the child was ready to be born—until Marina was ready to talk—she could do no more than keep her patient comfortable.

"Has anyone threatened you?" Olympia inquired.

She could barely hear the muffled reply. "No."

"Or you've had an uninvited guest, perhaps a suitor?"

Marina looked up, fixing reddened by innocent eyes on Olympia. "Only my family and some friends have come. They're trying to help. But it's hopeless!"

Olympia lowered her eyes. *Well, what now?* There was a possibility she hadn't considered. "This has something to do with your late husband."

Again, the reply was barely audible. "Yes."

"Ah!" said Olympia. "Have you—" But as soon as the words were out, she checked herself. She'd wanted to ask if Marina had any information about her husband's killer, but that could not be—not if the lady wanted the utmost secrecy.

Marina studied the floor for a while. "I was planning to give his clothes to the poor," she said at last, wiping her eyes. "It wouldn't have happened if the servants hadn't been so clumsy."

Olympia startled. "What wouldn't have—"

"I never knew him at all. I always wondered why we weren't closer."

Olympia grabbed Marina's elbow and looked her in the eye. "What is this? Were you estranged?"

"No. We got along for people living under the same roof, but—"

"But he was your husband!"

"I think I mentioned that he was always so preoccupied, so secretive."

"You did. Now, what else—"

Marina turned away, wiping a strand of dark hair from her face. "I don't think you'd understand."

Olympia raised a fair eyebrow. "Why not?"

"Because you're...a maiden."

"Oh. Well, I might understand more than you think." Which was true. And now she understood where this conversation was leading.

"For the last two years he's had nothing to do with me."

"Ah." In some compartment in the back of her mind, a key turned in the lock. "And you did not consent to

340

this…arrangement?"

"It was not even discussed."

Olympia frowned. *And you didn't think to speak up.* "Well! That's bad enough, of course, but there must be something else you wanted to tell me. Something that's happened since I last saw you."

Marina stared at the far wall. Then, fighting her exhaustion, she struggled to her feet. Olympia steadied her.

"This morning," said Marina, "I had the servants fetch my husband's chests from his storeroom. They banged them around more than necessary. Inside one of them, a cedar panel got knocked loose. It concealed…this!" She tottered over to the bed, extracted a cracked folded piece of parchment from beneath the mattress, and gave it to Olympia. "Here! The words aren't his, but it's in his hand."

Olympia unfolded the parchment. Tiny, painstakingly neat writing covered both sides of the page. The language was archaic, with some odd noun and verb endings. But these were hardly the document's most remarkable features. *"Kyrie eleison!"* she exclaimed, when she'd read only a third of the first side. "What is this?"

Wringing her hands, Marina faced her. "You must have a good idea. Could he have planned to use this…as evidence?"

With regret, Olympia threw back her head in denial. "In that case, he would have turned it over to the Post."

"I know." Marina slumped over, about to collapse.

Olympia braced her and made her sit. *Mother of God,* she prayed silently. *What shall I do?*

At that moment, someone wrapped on the door—

presumably the maid Christina.

"Come in," said Olympia, opening the door.

Christina, accompanied by the eunuch Damian came in, carrying a pitcher of hot water, as well as a tray of cups and utensils. They set them on the table.

"Thank you," said Olympia.

As soon as the servants had bowed and departed, Olympia closed the door. She took her apothecary box from her bag, and picked a handful of something from one compartment. This she dropped into the pitcher and stirred. "This is an herb from Cathay," she said, "called *tsai,* or something of the sort. It's as common with their people as wine is with ours. But it invigorates."

After a few moments, she poured some of the reddish-brown liquid into a clay cup, then added a generous spoonful of honey. "Here," she said, offering it to Marina. "Please drink this."

Olympia observed the woman as she sipped the liquid, cautious of its unfamiliar taste. Nevertheless, she seemed calmer.

Finally, Olympia summoned all her courage. "I know I promised to keep this a secret, and I still intend to. But considering what we've found, there's one other person we should tell."

Marina sat up straight. Her hair was loose, her eyes wide with fear. "You promised! Not the Logothete of the Dromos! Not the Varangians!"

Olympia clasped her hand. "No, not they. I said you could trust me. The person I have in mind is different. He'll

know what to do. He will act with the greatest discretion
and compassion because he's been in trouble himself."

Chapter 41

The knock on Michael's door came in the middle of the night, rousing him from a profound and dreamless sleep. At first, he ignored the racket, but the nuisance continued.

He groaned. He'd never get back to sleep. "Yes?"

"Master, there's a message for you."

It was George, with news from the Palace, no doubt. What could have happened in the last few hours?

Earlier, Michael had returned to the Guards' quarters after visiting Tripsychos. He then reviewed the facts of Bourtzes's case with the Akoluthos, but to no avail. Finally, the Varangian dismissed him. "You might as well go home and get some sleep."

Michael had not argued. Though he knew that the Akoluthos must be disgusted with him, he couldn't continue his quest without respite.

But now, in the dead of night, he forced himself out of bed. As soon as he'd opened the door, George thrust in a small scroll. "A private person delivered it. He's waiting downstairs."

"A private person? Waiting?" Michael cut the wax seal with his thumbnail, then cried out in joy and terror. *She* had reentered his life, though perhaps not in the way he wished. So, she was at Bourtzes's—doing what? What could be so important? "Quick! My horse!"

§

Olympia made good use of the time before Michael arrived. She went from Marina's room to Bourtzes's and lit the lamps, started a fire in the brazier, and began a search. But as soon as she heard a stirring in the lower regions of the house, she headed for the staircase.

Her pulse quickened. Whatever happened, she would do her duty—both to the truth and to Marina. But now, for good or ill, she would see Michael.

She heard his firm step on the stairwell, then on the landing. Finally he mounted the final flight of stairs, his head bowed, his dark hair spilled in his eyes.

"Michael?"

He looked up. His voice was barely audible. "Olympia!" He bounded up the next few steps, then hesitated. What if she rejected him still?

The fine hair above her upper lip glistened in the lamplight. He tried to commit this and every other detail of her face to memory...in case he saw her for the last time.

She continued her descent but paused on the step above him. She took both his hands in his and felt his sinews grow taught. Shaking, she drew a breath.

"Michael, I'm asking to forgive me...for what I said Monday. I understand now...I was wrong."

"You mean—"

"I was cruel to both of you. She sought me out this afternoon. I can see that she's a good woman."

"Barbara?" Still, he didn't dare hope...

"And I can see that I was not wrong about you, when I said I saw something in you."

"Well, we all sin, or most of us."

"I should not have been angry. Your sin was not against me. Well, I should not have been angry in any case."

"Lady, I would forgive any sin of yours."

"But I have never known a man."

"I promise—that would not matter."

"Oh? Well, now—for *my* sins, my father is trying to find me a husband."

"And that's none of your doing. Actually, your teacher warned me of that."

"Really?"

He reached out and cupped her cheek. "He did. And—"

"Ahem!"

The voice came from below. They sprung apart and coughed to cover their embarrassment.

Michael looked back, towards the landing, and saw the same tall, polite eunuch who had admitted him.

"Yes, Damian," said Olympia, straightening her headgear with feigned nonchalance. "Everything's under control here. You may be excused until His Honor is ready to leave." She watched until the fellow had retreated around the corner.

Michael gazed at her. "I was going to give him marching orders, but you got rid of him. Nothing perturbs you, does it?"

"I wouldn't say that. But as a doctor, I'll need to preserve my composure in every possible situation."

"Indeed."

She smiled significantly. "But hold! We must put aside all…personal concerns now. We have a serious problem. When you hear what she found…"

She further explained as they mounted the stairs to Marina's room. After she had made the introductions, she bolted the door and directed Michael to one of the chairs.

The widow, he noticed, was slumped on a bench made comfortable with pillows. Olympia refilled Marina's cup— "Medicine," she explained to Michael—and took a seat opposite her.

"You might want to search the deceased's belongings later," she said to Michael, "but I think we've found what's truly significant." She picked up the parchment.

Michael turned to Marina. "Lady, may I—"

She looked away. "I can't allow this. I recognized your name. You're in charge of the murder investigation. You'll go straight to the authorities."

Michael leaned towards her. "No, I won't. I wish neither to besmirch your husband's reputation, nor to cause you pain. But if I'm to help both you and the Empire, I must know all the facts."

Marina faced him again. "How can I trust you?"

Michael thought for a few moments, seeking the right approach before he replied. "You trust Lady Olympia because she's a physician and has an oath of confidentiality. You can consider me another sort of doctor—one who tries to heal the ills of the State."

Olympia nodded. But she knew that sometimes physicians had to cut off putrefied limbs in order to save the patient. Likewise, sometimes the authorities had to...remove traitors, the Empire's rotten members. Would Marina carry the analogy that far?

"Could I see this...writing now," Michael asked, observing the widow's timid expression. "I give my word that I'll hold my peace."

Slowly Marina's mouth formed the answer: "Yes."

Olympia passed Michael the document.

The room became so quiet that only the crackling of the parchment was audible. Several minutes elapsed before Marina spoke again, dabbing at her eyes with a handkerchief. "It's madness, isn't it? Wickedness!"

Michael studied the minute script that covered both sides of the page. "This is your husband's handwriting?"

"Yes, only much smaller than usual."

Because he wanted to make this text easy to conceal! "But the language is not his," said Michael. "And the words are not his, at least not originally."

"That's what I thought," said Marina.

"This text is ancient," said Michael and began to read it aloud. "'In the beginning was the Kingdom of Light, in which was God in his light and power and wisdom, abiding in His five dwellings of Sense, Reason, Thought, Imagination, and Intention. In the beginning was also the Kingdom of Darkness: the vile, the material, and the begotten—the dominion of the Lord of the Dark and his Archons.'"

"'It came to pass that the creatures of darkness increased and multiplied exceedingly, and their spawn entered the realm of Light.' Well!" Michael smoothed the document and set it on his lap. "I think you know what we have here."

"The language is ancient," said Olympia, "and it expresses an atrocious doctrine."

Marina glanced first at her, then at Michael. "It's heresy, isn't it?"

"Yes. Now, what do you know about the Bogomils?"

348

asked Olympia.

"They live in our westlands, don't they? They believe that the devil made man, and they do many evil things."

Olympia nodded. "They live not only in our westlands, but here in the Capital. Did any such people ever call upon your husband?"

"Not to my knowledge." Marina lowered her eyes and wept again. "He kept only the most respectable company, Palace officials and such."

Thinking of certain "respectable" people, Michael arched an eyebrow. Then he spoke. "I don't think this text is, strictly speaking, a Bogomil document, though certainly it's dualist. As Lady Olympia pointed out, the language is ancient. It contains some obsolete grammatical forms. In fact, …" Frowning, he read on. "Listen! 'This is the teaching of Manes, Apostle of Jesus Christ: the King of Darkness begot Adam.' What we have here is a classic Manichean text, or a condensation of several…although Manes was most certainly not an Apostle of Jesus Christ."

Marina clutched at her garment. "Alas, what am I to believe? What did my husband want with this?"

"Such things are copied in secret," said Michael, "for obvious reasons. However, Bourtzes could have turned it up in the course of his many travels in the service of the Empire. But the question remains—why did he hide it—and keep it?"

"He couldn't have been holding it as evidence, could he?" Marina's voice was low and resigned.

She made Michael want to weep. "That's not likely, my Lady."

"*Kyrie eleison!* He was a heretic, then, and a traitor to the Empire." She buried her face in her hands and began to sob long, choking sobs.

Immediately, Olympia was beside her, drawing her into an embrace. Michael stood up as well, and watched them in silence, until Marina's sobs grew fainter.

He began to pace the floor. "Let us consider. Most likely Bourtzes was not a Bogomil, though he sympathized with them. But their faith was too provincial and plebeian for him. He preferred something more high-toned, like classical Manicheism."

Marina snuffled. "Why did he— He was a good man, a hero."

Olympia patted Marina on the back and cast a significant glance at Michael.

"As for Lady Marina's concern that her husband was a traitor," he said, "I'm not so sure."

"How can he not be?" asked his widow.

Michael stopped pacing and looked down at his boots. "He was an upright man—that we know. But we also know that he was outraged by evil in high places. He disapproved of Saponas, and what could he have thought of the Imperial family, of their private lives? And let's bear in mind that he was an agent of the Post, and a well-traveled one at that. No doubt he saw vice and wickedness in low places also— everywhere—and no ray of hope for the future."

"So, he may have come to believe that the devil or the dark god made the world," Put in Olympia.

Marina groaned. "And so, he betrayed us. Now his memory will be desecrated. Alas, he deserves no better, but—"

Olympia hugged her. "Listen, we promised to keep this a secret, and we'll find a way."

Michael stood before them. "There *is* a way, and I don't think he was a traitor."

Marina spoke in a hushed voice. "How can you say that?"

"As for this document," Michael replied, "I believe that the three of us are the only ones who know of its existence. There's a community of Bogomils here in the City, and we just arrested one of them on a criminal charge. He has named all the members of his group, and your husband was not among them. He knows nothing of your husband, except for his name."

Marina breathed deeply.

"Also, your husband wrote in his last official report that he pretended to be a Bogomil while he was in Philippopolis. That's how we can explain away any—ah—suspicions that might arise. So, no one need know of this," he added, holding up the parchment.

Marina wiped her eyes. "You're not telling me. *Was* he a traitor?"

"I don't believe so. As I said, I know what was in his last report—which arrived here two days after his death. I didn't doubt his sincerity. However…" He winced, astonished that someone's duplicity could wound him so.

"Of course," said Olympia, "his words aren't enough by themselves."

"But if we consider them in the light of the facts, we can better evaluate them," continued Michael. "Let's consider his mission to Philippopolis. He disguised himself as an Imperial silk-goods merchant, and, as he said, 'pretended' to be a Bogomil in order to win the confidence of the local members of the sect."

"In other words, he put himself in great danger," added Olympia. "But what if he were...working for both sides?"

Michael nodded. He'd considered that possibility himself. "Still, he was risking his life. And let's recall that he infiltrated the rebel Tornicius's camp. Then he was also in grave danger. And what did he stand to gain by running that risk? Certainly, his only motive was the good of the Empire."

Now dry-eyed, Marina faced him. "But what if he were working for Tornicius as well? How can I believe that anything he did was what it seemed?"

Michael bowed his head. Alas, was anything more dreadful than betrayal? Bourtzes had sown the tainted seeds of doubt in all their minds. But though Michael needed to learn the whole truth, no one besides the three of them had to know the depth of Bourtzes's fall.

"Wait—" put in Olympia. "What of his investigation of the Patzinaks? He accused that noble of theirs..."

Michael looked up at her. "Metiga—yes. He suspected that that Metiga brought marauders over the Danube ice, but he lacked the evidence to prove it. Now, that mission brought your husband neither advantage, nor glory, but only an enemy."

Marina gasped. "Did this Metiga kill him?"

"He couldn't have, "said Michael. "A witness claims that he and his half-brother were dead drunk, in the back room of a tavern, around the time of the murder."

"But who can say what Bourtzes thought or intended," Olympia mused aloud. "Who can ever see into the human heart?"

Lately Michael had pondered that question himself. Somehow Father Zosimas felt that Saponas had the capacity for repentance, for belief. But Michael could not see it.

On the other hand, Michael knew he had only to look within himself to find a maelstrom of impulses and motivations: noble, bold, base, cowardly, vile. So, it must be with everyone. Still, everyone possessed a will, and the ability to vanquish this inner chaos, at least for a time. One could make conscious choices and take conscious risks. "We have yet to mention the main evidence in Bourtzes's favor—he's dead!"

The two women flinched, then nodded in understanding.

"So, who could have killed him—and why?"

"His former associates," Marina replied. "Heretics—the ones he knew, or the ones he 'pretended' with. They found him out—that he'd rejected his past life. They killed him to conceal their crimes."

Michael sighed. "Yes, but it seems that he had no contact with this local group of Bogomils. And there's also the possibility that someone in the government believed he was a heretic and a traitor and eliminated him in order to save the State both embarrassment and expense." He clutched his head. "A government official—someone like the Logothete of the Dromos."

Marina's eyes widened. "The Logothete of the

Dromos?"

"Yes, I've always suspected him, but earlier I didn't understand his possible motive."

A crease appeared between Olympia's eyebrows. "Indeed, why would the Logothete deal with Bourtzes's treason in that way. Why wouldn't he simply have arrested and interrogated the man?"

"That would make more sense," Michael replied, "unless the Logothete himself were involved in a plot and later changed his mind. But I don't want to believe that."

Olympia mumbled, "Of course." A taught silence followed her words.

After a long pause, Michael spoke. "Let's suppose that Bourtzes died because he knew too much—presumably about the conspiracy he described in his report. Let's suppose that at some time—most likely before he left for Philippopolis—he decided to renounce his double-mindedness and serve the Empire alone. And finally, let us believe his last words—that the Bogomils had infiltrated the provincial administration and hoped to secede from the Empire. But if he were on the track of something there, why didn't he stay to see things through. Why did he come running back to the City when there was no date set for his return?"

"If he were in danger there—" Olympia began.

"Yes," said Michael, "but whatever the man was—God rest his soul—he was no coward."

"Then why *did* he return?" asked Marina.

"Think!" said Michael. "No one has ever explained that—or how his killer knew just where to find him...

Wait!" He clutched his hand to his brow. "What if he returned at that time because he'd made an appointment before he left? And what if the person he arranged to meet was a fellow conspirator, whom he now planned to turn over to the authorities. And—most importantly—what if that person discovered that Bourtzes had changed sides...and killed him?"

Marina trembled. "But why didn't he arrest the man that night? If he'd asked for reinforcements—"

"I suspect he was laying a trap," said Michael. "He wanted to catch the culprit, or culprits, in the act. No doubt this assignation was simply a routine meeting in an oft—used place, perhaps in that abandoned barn. No doubt he planned to give his erstwhile confederate a much-adulterated report of his activities, and then arrange another rendezvous, at which he extract promises or evidence of men, money, or other aid from the plotters. He would implicate them while he had spies—reinforcements—concealed within earshot."

Marina regarded him sorrowfully. "But even alone, my husband could have defended himself against one man—against more than one!"

Michael exhaled in exasperation. "That's a difficulty I'm well aware of. But there's no evidence that he fought anyone face to face."

"Your latest interpretation makes Bourtzes quite devious," said Olympia, "though you're probably right."

Michael cleared his throat. "A man in Bourtzes's position had to be devious although we might prefer to use the word 'resourceful.'"

The widow snuffled loudly.

Michael nodded towards her. "Forgive me, Lady." He watched her for a moment, relaxing when he saw her dab at her nose and put her handkerchief away. "Of course, there's one thing wrong with my explanation: how did the killer learn that Bourtzes had changed sides?"

"How indeed," asked Olympia.

Michael sat, and rested his chin in his hands, his elbows on his knee. He closed his eyes in thought. His mind was like a night landscape illumined by a lightning flash. In an instant he saw all the facts of the case, and enlightenment struck him.

He blinked, then jumped up. "God help us if they've escaped!... Excuse me, ladies, I must go. If only I'm not too late!"

Olympia also rose. "What is it? Who?-—"

Michael's gaze did not meet hers but turned inward, confronting a new and terrible sight. He spoke in a whisper. "According to the old adage, one can tell a lion by his claws. But the lion has been lying beside us all this time, and we didn't even know him."

Chapter 42

Ragged, blackish clouds scudded across the night sky. As Michael galloped his horse down the deserted Mese, cold air whipped his face. Monuments, arches, and walls winged past him. Suddenly the curved tiers of the Hippodrome loomed ahead. Across the street rose the squarish bulk of the Pretorium, home of all municipal offices.

This was his first stop. "We need help," he said, shoving his signet ring under the night guard's nose. After explaining exactly what sort of help was required, he swung into the saddle again. Only when he reached the Augusteum did he slow his mount to a walk, looking warily around him. He reined in and dismounted before a postern in the Palace wall.

"Taronites here!" He rapped on the thick, iron-bound door, then heard a stirring on the battlements above him. If he were an enemy, he thought, he could expect an arrow in the chest. Instead, the narrow gate creaked open. Two burly Varangians in chain mail guarded it.

"I need to see the Akoluthos," said Michael.

"He's probably asleep," said one of the guards.

"I need to speak with him immediately."

The other guard scratched his stubby beard in bewilderment. "What's wrong?"

"Bourtzes's killer. I've—"

"Come in."

A third Varangian arrived, and escorted Michael and his horse to the Varangians' headquarters. At the office of the

Akoluthos, he instructed Michael, "Now wait," and led away his horse.

Michael groaned in dismay. *Wait?* He had no choice. He entered the anteroom and slumped on a bench, trying to rub the weariness from his eyes. The yellow flame in a hanging lamp sputtered. Outside the arched windows, shadows of night lay over the courtyard.

Did he sleep? He knew nothing until someone called his name: "Michael!"

Coming awake, he opened his eyes. Father Zosimas was standing over him.

Michael sprang up and kissed the monk's hand. "Please, have a seat," he said, indicating the bench. "I thought you'd gone back to the monastery."

"I did, very briefly. But the Abbot gave me his blessing to return; he felt I might accomplish something here. Well, I did visit Saponas in his cell. When the guards chased me out, I slept in the narthex of the Church of the Savior—at least until the commotion woke me up. I learned that you were here."

"So you visited Saponas."

"He wanted me to come."

Michael snorted. "I never considered you naïve."

"Naïve?" Zosimas's eyes widened. "I assure you—I'm not."

"Why do you think he wants to speak with you? He's trying to make a good impression on the authorities so that they'll treat him leniently."

"Michael! He's a deeply troubled man, and I know he expects no mercy."

"As you'll recall, he *did* kill someone."

"Yes, and I know he tried to kill you."

"Well, the man has so many sins on his soul," said Michael. "He's no saint. So, what do you expect from him?"

"He can always repent."

Again, Michael snorted.

"Think! Beneath his buffoonery is his pain, and beneath his pain is...the inner man."

"The inner man needs a bath."

"Of course. The mirror must be cleaned and polished before it can give a true reflection...and, Michael..."

"Yes?"

"A saint is not someone who has no sins. There is no man without sin, save One only. But rather a saint is someone who, despite his sins, turns to God and cleaves to him, who stays so close that the Divine Light shines in him."

Michael swallowed awkwardly. "I see." He felt that another sarcastic remark would be out of place.

"You know," said the monk, "Saponas is also willing to discuss the Bogomil faith.

Forgetting his resolution, Michael raised an eyebrow. "Please! Don't tell me you've converted him."

Zosimas cleared his throat. His faint, now uneasy smile was half-hidden in his beard. "No, but whatever he is, or will be, he needs a friend... In any case, I've tried to explain to him that there are not two opposing gods, but One, who created nothing for evil. Only man's abuse of food, drink, and the like is evil."

"I daresay he knows about that first hand."

The monk furrowed his brow. "Michael, please!... We also talked about free will and the Fall. Man may have a propensity for wickedness, but he's still made in God's image. He's hardly as bad as the dualists think, or certain Latin writers."

"Did Saponas believe what you said?"

"He listened. He admits, of course, that a good God would create nothing evil."

"But he still believes in two gods." Michael placed a hand on Zosimas's forearm. "Forgive me for taunting you. But I simply cannot imagine that wily jester correcting himself."

"One can't give up hope, you know. Even *he* hasn't, in spite of himself."

"Just don't let him fool you."

Zosimas laughed softly. "I won't."

Michael hung his head. He should know better: if anyone could fathom the depths of the human heart, it was Father Zosimas. "I'm sorry I'm so cynical. And you...if you can understand Saponas, I think you'll understand what I learned from Bourtzes's widow tonight. I know you'll tell no one."

"Yes," Zosimas concluded, after hearing the details of Michael's discovery, "you and Lady Olympia acted wisely. And I'm pleased to hear that you've put things right between you."

Michael nodded.

"And we must continue to pray for Bourtzes's soul."

Michael blinked. Had the light in the room changed? It seemed brighter, though the single oil lamp was still flickering.

But now a distant commotion caught Michael's attention: a stirring and rustling within the Akolouthos's office, then the sound of a bolt sliding.

"Well," he said, patting his side to make certain he had his dagger. "The Akoluthos is here. Now we'll arrest Bourtzes's murderers."

At once, Zosimas was on his feet. "I'll come with you, son."

"No! I mean—I'm sorry, but you can't go where I'm going. It will be dangerous."

"Can't I?" There was a distant look in his blue eyes. "But you stood by me during my trial."

"Of course I did, but I was able to help—" Michael choked on his words; they were all wrong. "Er—I would have given you moral support even if I could not testify or conduct my own investigation. I would have—"

The monk reached up and laid a hand on Michael's shoulder. "Oh, I know I'm a useless old man—"

Again, before Michael gasped in horror, he noticed the shifting light in the room. Was the lamp burning brighter? "But you're not old!"

"Oh, but I am. And to tell the truth, I've found the past two weeks invigorating. I've also realized how much I've placed my hopes on you, as though you were my own son. Some people might censure me for such an attachment, but—"

"How could they?"

"Come now. I'm a monk. I should be above all earthly ties. Still, I won't ignore the bond between us. I..." A smile flitted across the fine lines of Zosimas's face. "I'll go back to the church now. If I can do no more than pray for you, so be it."

§

Lagging behind the ranks of Varangians in jangling chain mail, Michael and the Akoluthos rode side by side, pacing their horses at a brisk trot. By the time they reached the pale, mountainous form of the Church of the Holy Apostles, the sky had lightened to the color of iron. The jagged outline of the ruined Wall of Constantine loomed before them.

Michael and his companion slowed their mounts to a walk, allowing the main body of the troops to charge ahead. Once they'd disappeared around a corner, Michael returned to the conversation he'd begun when the Akoluthos appeared in his office. "So you see, they tried—successfully for a while—to throw us off the scent. They stole all but Bourtzes's small coins so it would appear that he had been robbed. They trampled on his cross so that we'd think the Bogomils killed him. But they went through his mail in earnest. They wanted to find his last report, to learn just how much he knew. But the report wasn't there to begin with, and, in any case, it did not explain everything."

The Akoluthos scowled. "I see now. It was a political crime. But also an act of violence—by two Patzinaks."

"A brutal act."

The Varangian swore in Norse, then in Russian, for a good minute or two, until they reached the turn-off the troops had taken. As they swung their mounts to the left, Michael looked back. "I see no one, but I'm certain I heard another horse behind us."

"What of it? With us you're safe."

When they reached the Inn of the Golden Fleece, mail-clad Varangians and militiamen in brief tunics milled around the entrance. The arched double doors themselves hung open, spilling yellow lamplight across the walk. In a far corner of the yard, cloaks and blankets covered several lumpy but unmistakably human forms.

An underofficer hurried towards the Akoluthos. "We've got the place surrounded, for all the good it's done."

"What do you mean?"

The Varangian motioned towards the covered bodies. "We've already lost some men. Also, they can't get out, but we can't get in. Before we got here, the militia sent in a couple of their people to break down the bastards' door. It seems they got in all right, but the earth must have swallowed them."

"Well!" said Michael. "Our suspects are certainly acting guilty."

The Akoluthos grunted, the addressed the officer again. "Has anyone else tried to storm their rooms?"

"No one's volunteered. But we've got men on the staircase. Um—we've already lost a few of those."

The Akoluthos scratched his beard in thought. "I don't know how we can get someone into their quarters without attracting their attention. He'd only share the fate of the militiamen."

"At least one of the Patzinaks is shooting out their window now," said the underofficer. "He's hit several of our men."

The Akoluthos scowled again and turned to Michael.

"Taronites, thank you for your help, But now you can tie your horse somewhere and do...I don't know what. The proprietor and his staff have barricaded themselves in the common room. You can join them or...just stay out of the way! My officers and I will find a way to flush them."

Michael didn't see how—nor how the Patzinaks could escape. He tethered his horse and surveyed the scene. He was like the rope of a catapult, wound to the limit.

He recalled that the culprits' rooms were on the second floor of the inn, on the left and to the rear. But the thick growth of trees—mostly pines—between the inn and the neighboring house, blocked his view of the windows.

All the more reason to get a better look, to go into the midst of the fray. Heart pounding, he threw his cloak back over his shoulders. He fingered the knife at his belt and started for the trees.

"Watch out, Taronites," called the Akoluthos. "You're not wearing armor." Then, as if catching sight of something out of the corner of his eye, he turned, staring back up the street. "Halt! Who're you?"

Michael followed his gaze. In the pre-dawn gloom, he saw—or thought he saw, a dark figure vanish into the shadows on the far side of the house next door.

Pleased that the Akoluthos was distracted, he gave the apparition no more thought; no doubt it was a drunkard or a lecher returning from his nocturnal revels.

Michael slipped around the corner of the inn and edged along the side of the neighboring house. Without taking his eyes from the inn, he passed between naked, twisted oak limbs and bushy pine branches.

"Down! Over here!"

Michael fell to his knees and crawled towards the voice. Concealed behind the dense, meshed branches of seedling trees and underbrush were several militiamen and Varangians. All had nocked arrows to their bows.

"They're up there." One of the Varangians nodded towards the wall of the inn, where a casement hung open, its glass panes shattered. "They're shooting through their back window too. Ho! Drop!"

They rose to a crouch. Michael brushed dirt and dry leaves from his clothes. The others didn't bother.

The Varangian indicated the black maw of the window. "They can see us, but we can't see a damn thing. We're shooting blind."

Michael set his lips. Though now the Patzinaks had the advantage, they could not hold out forever. Sooner or later, they'd run out of arrows.

Suddenly Michael heard a rustle, and the crackle of underbrush somewhere behind the inn. He looked towards the whitish bulk of the stables. Missiles whined back and forth, thunking into tree trunks, bouncing off walls. Someone near the stables emitted an agonizing shriek.

One of the Varangians swore. "Our men were told to stay behind the stables."

"They can hardly see their target from there," said Michael.

"No, but they won't get killed, either. And nobody will get past them."

"I wonder."

Someone yelled another warning, and they dropped to

their bellies again. More bolts whined overhead. Then there were more groans, more footsteps, more commotion around the Patzinaks's rear window.

Somewhere closer to hand, an inhuman howl rent the air.

A militiaman whispered to his comrades. "What happened? Did we get one?"

Yes, thought Michael. Unless—

For a short while, all was silent. Then one arrow after another hissed overhead. Michael waited, trembling, for the stillness he expected. When he could hear no more than the breeze in the branches, he raised himself to his hands and knees. His companions still lay flat.

Fox-like, he crept towards the stables, pulling himself to his feet behind a scrub oak with a few tattered leaves clinging to it. From here he could see the back wall of the inn, where, one story up, another shattered casement hung open. There was no movement there, no change in the light.

Then he caught sight of the rope dangling from a huge oak between the window and the stables. He was not in the least surprised.

His eyes followed the still-swaying rope from its free end up to the slip-knot around a broken limb. No one could have hidden in the oak's bare crown.

But just beyond it rose two huge pines, their upper branches a dense green. Heart pounding, Michael moved towards them—close, too close!

"Aiii!" A familiar stench filled the air. Something fell upon him, knocking him to the ground. Then it hauled him up, pinning his arms to his sides with the force of iron bands. He fumbled for his knife but found the sheath empty.

"You die!" rasped his captor.

Michael could feel edge of the blade against his neck, high on the right. He recognized the gut-churning stink of sweat and horses. So, which Patzinak was it? He twisted, hoping to cast a glimpse, and felt the desperate man move the blade up to his windpipe.

"Bastards!" The Patzinak's voice was high and reedy. "I got your man! You let me go, or I kill him."

Michael recognized his voice. He tried to speak, but the pressure on his throat choked him, and he gasped for breath. Now even foul air was sweet.

The Varangians' faint voiced drifted towards him on the breeze. No doubt they were agreeing to let the wretch go, in order to save Michael's life.

But Michael doubted that the assassin would spare him under any circumstances.

Finally, the Patzinak lowered the knife. Once more his grip spanned Michael's chest and upper arms. He backed past the stables—where no Varangians now stood guard— towards the hedgerow behind it.

Michael drew a deep breath. He had to get the villain talking; it might increase his chances of survival. "Good morning, Uzun, so-called brother of Metiga."

"He dead."

"You're no brother of his, and our men didn't kill him. You did."

"Who care who kill him."

"I do—because the two of you killed Bourtzes." He paused for breath. "No doubt you envied Metiga's position and prestige." Again, he gulped down air. "But you had one thing in common. You were both working with the Bogomils."

The Patzinak forced Michael further back, towards the hedgerow, and Michael swallowed yet another breath. "You were in the westlands...in Philippopolis, before you came here."

"I see that sheep-fornicator there. He say to everyone he was a merchant."

"You mean...Bourtzes."

"I not know Bourtzes, but why that sonofabitch the under-general come visit him? Ha! He don't fool me!"

Stalling for time, Michael corrected him. "That's Naum Vladislavich, *hypostrategos* of the theme." He fell silent because his throat and chest ached. Well, good! he thought. He was making the Patzinak angry. Maybe he would talk more freely now—if he didn't kill Michael first.

"So, I know something's up, and I run for Constantinople."

It was just as Michael thought. Uzun could have made the trip in almost as little time as a State courier. Instead of post horses, he would have used those provided by his fellow tribesmen in the area. "You told Metiga that someone from the Capital had found you out. When you described the man, he knew it was Bourtzes, because Bourtzes was supposedly plotting with him."

"The bastard double-cross him!"

"You didn't spare Bourtzes, did you?" No doubt the Patzinak had a similar fate in store for Michael.

Michael's career, which seemed most promising now

that he'd found the murderers, would be cut short. Olympia would be forced to marry a man of her father's choice. And Michael would die before he was ready; he was still young, with countless foibles and outright sins, and he had left so much undone.

And besides, it must be excruciating to have one's throat cut, worse to be raped.

But he wouldn't die until he'd learned the whole truth.

Though his throat was parched, he forced himself to speak. "So, you two plotted to kill Bourtzes." Let Uzun brag a little. "I can guess how you did it."

The Patzinak grunted a reply. Watching a Varangian archer on the stable roof, he changed his direction and backed Michael into a stand of trees.

Now Michael feared he'd learn no more.

His head spun. Was he already dead? The dry, needle-covered dirt below, the lightening sky above him tilted, the receded, around him.

He saw himself as a fifteen-year-old, sitting in a high-ceilinged Palace schoolroom. Psellus, the distinguished teacher, was explaining Plato's allegory of the cave. Had Michael come out into the sunlight? Would he know the Mystery hidden from all the ages?

Above him, pinkish wisps of clouds streaked the sky—but where was he? Even in his present abode, in this strange place beyond the world, something broke the silence; he could hear the soft crunch of leaves and pine needles behind him. He felt another presence—very close—and sensed a faint, bittersweet smell.

"Take your hands off him at once!" The newcomer's

voice was soft and very familiar.

"Aiii!" Uzun pushed Michael away and spun around. "Piss off, dog!" He howled again, as if he'd just seen a horrific steppe demon.

Michael hit the ground. His side stung, but he staggered to his feet in time to take in everything: Uzun hurling himself upon the dark-clad newcomer; the supine form of the monk; Uzun running, his black hair streaming behind him; then a deadly thrum, a high shriek, and Uzun spilling on his face, an arrow shaft vibrating in his back.

Moaning, Michael dropped to his knees beside Father Zosimas. He wished he could yell like the Patzinak, yell until his cry echoed against the vault of the heavens.

The monk still lived. His blue eyes were clear. "Michael, *chaire,* rejoice!" he began, but his greeting ended in an obscene gurgle.

Rejoice? thought Michael. He saw why Zosimas spoke with difficulty: a familiar dagger hilt—Michael's own— protruded from the monk's chest.

Michael reached for it, then stopped himself. Better to leave that for a doctor.

Instead, he took Zosimas's hand in his. "Why did you follow me? I told you—" He broke off, choking back a sob.

"Remember the day...you came to visit me in the scriptorium?"

"Yes." Warm tears coursed down Michael's cheeks.

"I said...I should have been a soldier. Now...a vain old man...has his wish. And it's you who can't come...where I'm going. I—" He broke off coughing and gasping. When he stopped, a pinkish foam covered his lips.

"No!" cried Michael, "don't try to talk." He recalled his foolish words of a few hours ago. Though his hands shook, he fumbled in his belt pouch for his handkerchief, then wiped Zosimas's mouth. "I'll get help. It will be all right." Frantically he searched the yard and saw two Varangians hurrying toward them.

Zosimas spoke in a hoarse whisper. "Michael—"

"Spare yourself!"

"I was glad to have these days with you. I watched over you…after Theodore was gone." He coughed again, bringing up bright blood that stained his light, graying beard. He drew a rasping breath.

"Don't talk!" said Michael.

"You can manage…by yourself—now." The monk's blue eyes still had the clear, active look of the living as he clasped Michael's hand in his. But almost at once, Michael felt his grip relax.

"He's gone," Michael cried out, hurling his grief, like a stone from a catapult, at the distant sun. Now he could weep. Now the taught ropes within him had gone slack.

And now the earth seemed to tremble beneath him. Like a drunkard with no control over his movements, he tried to will his actions. This I must do! he thought, between ragged sobs. He folded the monk's hands on his beast, then closed his eyes. Then he could do no more. He slumped over and buried his face in the rough, sticky cloth of Zosimas's habit, his tears mingling with the blood.

Chapter 43

After what seemed an eon but what must have been the twinkling of an eye, Michael noticed the tramp of boots behind him. He turned as several Varangians approached. "Taronites!" said the officer. "We'll take care of everything. But now Metiga is dying. You must get his confession."

Slowly, Michael rose to his knees and shook his head. Metiga? Who was he?... Ah! he remembered. To be sure, Uzun did leave certain questions unanswered.

"Uzun told me that Metiga was dead," Michael remarked, as a Varangian helped him to his feet.

"He will be soon. So hurry!"

Michael cast a backward glance at Zosimas, but the Varangians urged him on. "Someone will stay with him. We called a priest and sent a messenger to the monastery."

Michael allowed them to guide them where they would. Putting one foot in front of the other was the most he could do.

After what seemed another eon, they entered the inn and ascended the stairs. On the second floor, muffled voices drifted towards him from behind a door hanging half on, half off its hinges. Moments later, a familiar strapping, mail-clad form appeared in the doorway.

"There you are!" The Akoluthos enfolded Michael in a bear hug, which made him feel alive once more.

"How did you get in here?" asked Michael.

The Akoluthos released him. "When the shooting stopped, we suspected something and mounted a second assault on their room. This time we got in—and found Metiga on the floor. Then someone told us that Uzun had been shot escaping, so we figured out the rest. Now come!"

Michael stepped into the room, gagging on the now-familiar Patzinak odor. In an instant, he took in the wreckage: overturned chairs, chests moved to hold the door shut, cups, arrows, broken glass, blood on the carpet. And, off to his left, two bodies in militiamen's clothes. One had a bowstring twisted around his neck, the other a gaping slit throat.

"Cover them," said Michael. "Now, where's Metiga?"

"In the bedroom. We found him by the window here, with a knife in his back!"

Metiga lay supine on one of the beds. His torso was bare, bandaged with strips no doubt cut from his good linen shirts. Blood soaked the bedclothes beneath him.

The Patzinak's almond-shaped eyes were half-closed. Michael wondered if he were conscious. "Metiga?"

"H-here." The Patzinak coughed, and a rivulet of blood ran down his chin.

"Who did this? Uzun?"

The Patzinak groaned. "While I was...at window," he said, then coughed again.

Michael waited until the spell had ceased, and a militiaman had wiped away the blood. "I'll do most of the talking. Just answer yes or no." Was it providential that things had turned out this way?

Metiga opened his eyes fully, and Michael read a reluctant agreement in their adamantine blackness. "You win...now."

"You and Uzun killed Bourtzes because he knew you were plotting against the Empire." Michael would have to be careful here; he could not reveal Bourtzes's secret. "So you trapped him at Bourtzes's meeting place with you—that old barn. Most probably, one of you threw a lasso around him."

The Akoluthos thumped his forehead with his fist. "Ha! So that's why he couldn't defend himself!"

"Yes," whispered Metiga.

"Who but the horse people have such skill with a rope?" asked Michael. "Even night can't hinder them."

The Varangians mumbled their approval.

"So, Metiga," Michael continued, "you two strangled him—most probably with a bowstring—and...ah...did the devil knows what else to him. You were enraged. Afterwards, you rearranged his clothes somewhat, to conceal your...misdeeds. You carried him to the beech grove and left him. Then you took his horse into the ruined barn, built a fire, and went through his saddlebags."

"Yes. The bastard—" Metiga's outburst cost him dearly; once again he coughed blood.

Now the Akoluthos broke in. "Taronites! How did they know where to find Bourtzes?"

Michael looked him straight in the eye. "Bourtzes made an appointment with Metiga before he left for Philippopolis. He was a provocateur. As he said in his last report, he was pretending to be a Bogomil."

The Akoluthos laughed. "Well, I'll be damned! What a trick! But how did those heathens do it? I thought they were dead drunk."

374

"They were playacting." Michael turned to Metiga again. The Patzinak's eyes were sinking, and the skin across his cheekbones looked thin and taut. He had little time left.

"You must have poured wine over your undergarments, so you'd reek of it," Michael continued. "You pretended to be drunk, so that the proprietor of the Golden Gryphon would put you to bed in the back room, where—to his knowledge—you slept until the middle of the night, when you got up and asked for more wine. But I know otherwise: during that time, you slipped out the window to meet Bourtzes."

"Yes," rasped Metiga. He squeezed his eyes shut, as if fighting pain.

"Were you also conspiring against Father Zosimas?"

"No. But we and...our friends...not like him." He closed his eyes.

"That's why I saw you at the tavern Monday noon. True, you had legitimate business at the Palace, but you came to the wine shop hoping to hear news of the trial."

The Akoluthos asked the next question. "Metiga, who are your friends?"

"The Bogomils of Philippopolis," said Michael. "And perhaps the Paulicians. Uzun was most probably their contact. The heretics wanted to secede from the Empire, but they couldn't do it on their own. They needed good fighters, like the Patzinaks."

Metiga opened his eyes again. "Yes."

"We know that the Mayor of Philippopolis was complicit," said Michael. "Tell me, did you set a date for your revolt?"

"No. Too soon."

"But, in any case, Bourtzes fooled you," said Michael. "Thank God for that!" He paused for breath. "Last winter, you incited Tirakh Khan's people to cross the Danube."

"Yes."

The Akoluthos swore.

"You win...now," said Metiga. "But someday..." He began to cough again.

"Not likely!" The Akoluthos took Michael by the elbow. "Let's go."

"Why?"

"He's dying, and it won't be pretty."

§

The Akoluthos and his men took Michael to the common room, once more open, and practically force-fed him bread and wine. After a while, he felt slightly more alive and slumped at the table.

He startled as the doors swung open, and the Logothete of the Dromos came in. He pulled up a chair next to Michael, and placed a hand on his shoulder. "Michael, I heard what happened. I'm sorry."

Michael bowed his head. "And I'm sorry—that I ever doubted you."

Blachernites snorted. "You were doing a thorough job. I can't complain about that."

"That's kind of you."

"As I said, I'm sorry about your monk. I was wrong about him, but knowing what I do of the world, I don't trust anyone. Well, you know what we've seen."

Michael grimaced, remembering what they had both

seen.

"But instead of a sinner, he turned out to be a saint," said the Logothete.

"A crazy one," the Akoluthos put in. "Though one couldn't ask for a braver man. If I had ten like him—"

"He was a good soldier of the Heavenly King," said Blachernites.

Michael did not reply, though he was glad at the Logothete's change of heart. He gazed through the windows of the common room. The shutters had been thrown open, and the sky was bright, the sun shining on the pinkish-white houses across the street. He lived, though he had felt the chill touch of death. He lived, though now his grief had nearly laid him in the grave. He lived, and the life that coursed through his veins was the same life that quickened the universe, filling all things with joy. Joy?…

"Eh, Michael?" the Logothete prompted him.

He startled. "Yes?"

"How did you find out about the Patzinaks?"

Michael raised an inner shield and looked his superior straight in the face. "You'll recall that Bourtzes, in his last dispatch, said he pretended to be a Bogomil when he was in Philippopolis. It took me a while to realize what he did not say. He was engaged in a complex provocation, playing the Bogomil traitor here in the City as well, in the process of laying a trap. If he had not been killed when he was, he would have told us more when the trap was in place."

The Logothete nodded.

"He too was a brave man," said Michael. "He exposed himself to great danger."

"As I asked, how did you settle on the Patzinaks?"

"Well, in the first place, although many people could have made an assignation with Bourtzes when he returned to the City, who but the Patzinaks had both the skill and the opportunity to dispatch him, under those circumstances?"

"But how did you settle on *those two?*"

"Saponas mentioned drinking with Uzun in a tavern on the Adrianople road, in a completely innocent encounter. Uzun was on his way to the City, and arrived here about a week before Bourtzes's death. He had been in the west country and had seen Bourtzes meeting with an official of the theme, thus concluding that the man was a traitor to their cause. Once Uzun arrived here, he made contact with Metiga. He identified himself to us as his brother, though we have no proof of that. It's analogous to the case of Peter of Serrhes and his so-called 'cousin.'"

"I see," said Blachernites, nodding briskly. "Then too, Uzun did kill Metiga, so most probably they were not brothers. Of course, these barbarians with their plural wives have no concept of family as we know it."

"But do we?" asked Michael. "We betray our wives, castrate our sons, force our daughters into marriage. And I have no doubt that if our brother got in our way, we'd kill him as well."

"Dear me!" said the Logothete. "Not everyone does such things. If they did, the Romans would die out. But we're none too virtuous. On the other hand, I'm sure that many Patzinaks, despite their strange customs, are decent folk who live without violence."

Michael shrugged. "All that matters is that these two

Patzinaks plotted against the Empire, and now they're dead."

Blachernites reached up and clapped Michael on the shoulder. "Quite so! Congratulations on a job well done."

A job well done indeed. Aside from himself, only two living people knew the whole truth.

Chapter 44

For Michael, the rest of the day passed in a haze of grief; he recalled being escorted home and put to bed. But the very next morning, he was summoned to the Palace to review the case with the Logothete of the Dromos and the Akoluthos and the Varangian guard. It was almost evening when they finished.

Without stopping to eat, Michael rode out to the Monastery of the Studion to visit Zosimas's bier. He entered the gates in the gathering dusk and approached the whitish, timber-roofed church. In the narthex, the Abbot, leaning on his staff, detained him.

"Perhaps I shouldn't have let Father Zosimas out of the monastery for more than a day," he said. "But I wanted to give him time to settle his case. Then too, though he did things that were unusual for a monk, he did only good. He rescued a man from torture, and he...saved your life."

Michael felt a lump in his throat. The Abbot patted him on the shoulder and departed.

Next Michael heard a rustling, and the inner door of the church swung open. Mother Anastasia, emerged, accompanied by two other nuns. She wiped her broad cheeks with a handkerchief and turned towards Michael. "I wanted to thank you for helping my brother."

Michael bowed his head; he felt tears coming on. "I could do no other, but it wasn't enough."

"I know you loved him," said the Abbess. "And listen— I can't be your mother—or your father—but if you ever need family, I'll be your aunt or your older sister."

"Thank you. I'll remember that."

She wiped her eyes again, then turned to her companions. "Come, it's time to return to the convent." The two nuns flanked her, supporting her.

The outside doors swung shut, and Michael turned back towards the church. A sob wracked him, and he wept silently, until a metallic clank caught his attention. He wiped his eyes with his sleeve, and as the inner doors swung open, he saw a stout form emerge from the nave, accompanied by two Varangians in red tunics.

It was Saponas, his hands and feet shackled, his garment soiled. In the fading light, his face looked sickly pale. "I saw him. The powers that be allowed it. Of course, they sent these bears along to guard me," he said, indicating the Varangians with a nod of his shaggy head. "I'll remember—he never condemned me."

Michael couldn't say the same for himself. "I know he did. I understand." He reached out and clapped Saponas on the shoulder. "Are they treating you well?"

"Well enough."

"I'll use my poor influence to make certain you're dealt with fairly." He bowed and stepped aside as Saponas, chains rattling, went out into the dark.

Finally, Michael summoned enough courage to enter the church. He walked up the elongated nave, illuminated by hanging lamps. The thick air was redolent of incense and beeswax.

The bier stood before the iconostasis, where the solemn faces of the saints, each surrounded by a nimbus of gold, kept watch.

A rack of candles stood to one side of the bier, while on the other, three monks gathered around a lectern. They took turns reading the Psalter, the words falling like a soft rain. "The Lord hear thee in the day of affliction; the name of the God of Jacob defend thee."

Michael knelt by the bier to pray and let his tears flow unrestrained. After what seemed an age, he stood and wiped his eyes. Father Zosimas was dressed in priestly vestments of gold-trimmed white. A liturgical veil, known as an *aer*, covered his face, and a Gospel book rested in his hands.

Was this still form the man that Michael had known, the man who had been a second father to him? Yes, he looked the same, but he was already far away.

The candles flickered, their light glistening on the silk and fine linen of Zosimas's garments. But, to Michael, the monk's beard, spread out on his chest like a silver cover, was finer than these.

Finally, Michael turned to go. Once more he traversed the length of the old-fashioned, elongated nave, his footsteps echoing against the dark timbers of the ceiling.

How would he carry on tonight, and tomorrow, and all the unnumbered days ahead of him? A good man and a friend had died, and Michael would not be comforted. Evil existed, and no explanation, not even of the sort that Father Zosimas had made to Saponas, would take away the pain. What good was all the talk of the revolt of Lucifer, the Fall, and free will? At the moment, none that Michael knew of.

But he had not forgotten the luminous sky of yesterday morning and his intuition of universal joy. It was a joy unknown to the Bogomils. No, he could not accept the solution that had tempted both Saponas and Bourtzes.

Bourtzes! Yes, Michael had another stop to make tonight.

Suddenly, chillled air gusted in from the back of the nave, and a growing murmur reached his ears. Someone had opened the outer doors.

Michael went out into the narthex and came face to face with the swarthy, sorrow-worn countenance of the Patriarch. A monk's veil covered his head, and his dark mantle swirled around him as the clergy who accompanied him closed the doors behind him.

"Michael!" The hard planes of his face softened.

Michael stepped forward to kiss his hand, but he passed his staff to a member of his retinue and embraced Michael quickly. "When I asked for your help, I never expected the matter to end like this."

"It's not your fault—not at all—but that's beside the point," the Patriarch said, releasing him. "'Now we've cleared him,' I thought. 'Now we'll make him a bishop.'"

"I don't think he wanted that."

The Patriarch slipped an arm around Michael's shoulders. "Oh, I know. He was too humble—ahem—if that's possible. If we ever meet in the next world, I'll ask him: 'Did you have to go to such lengths to avoid the episcopate?'"

Michael blinked back a tear. "You know he didn't. He never did anything with calculation. But I can't help wondering: did he know he'd — ? Did he know I'd...need him?"

"Perhaps. He was a more perfect man than either of us.

Who can say what he knew?"

§

Michael arrived at Bourtzes's house late, around the hour of Compline. A wooden gong sounded in the distance.

Tonight he found Marina—and Olympia—sitting on the couch in the lady's room. And tonight the widow, though still pale and red-eyed, appeared stronger.

He sank into a chair opposite them. "You can rest assured," he told Marina, "that your husband's reputation is safe. The Court officials believe that His Honor was pretending to be a Bogomil in order to entrap heretics and traitors—which is true. And as far as the Court is concerned, when he returned to the City, he was laying a snare for Metiga and Uzun—which is also true. But the Patzinaks had learned that he was double-dealing, and so they killed him."

"Truly?"

"Truly. So, as far as they're concerned, Bourtzes is a hero, which is exactly what we wish."

"But you are also a hero," said Marina, "and a brilliant man."

"Oh, come now!" Michael found the lady's adulation embarrassing. No doubt she'd lavished the same sort of admiration on Bourtzes, and it had done her no good.

"You deserve all the credit they give you," said Olympia.

"Much of it is yours, Ol—Er, Lady..." Michael coughed to cover his loss and felt his cheeks burn.

If Olympia noticed, she didn't let on. "Some aspects of this case are still unclear to me. First of all, was Saponas cooperating with the Patzinaks?"

384

"Not at all, though I'm sure they welcomed his disruptive activities. Of course, Saponas will still be tried for murder and conspiracy—possibly for treason, though he'll probably be treated with clemency."

"What makes you think that?"

Michael took a deep breath. "I learned that Father Zosimas—God rest his soul—bent the ear of almost every official in the Palace—he even got in to see the Emperor. Father Zosimas believed that Saponas was repentant or that he would repent."

"So, he'll probably be exiled, imprisoned in a fortress on the Princes' Islands. And I understand that Father Jonas, who brought accusations against Father Zosimas, will end up in the same place. He'll be under house arrest in a monastery there."

"Like the Publican and the Pharisee," said Olympia.

They nodded and fell silent. A coal in the brazier popped. Somewhere in the house, a beam creaked.

It was Olympia who broke the silence. "Another question: last winter Bourtzes accused Metiga of bringing Tirakh Khan's people over the ice. What is the truth of the matter?"

"Whether Bourtzes actually knew or not, Metiga *did* incite Tirakh to cross the river. He admitted it before he died. He and Tirakh were actually on the same side, sowing disruption."

"Ah!" said Olympia.

"But enough of that. Let me explain how I—we—established the Patzinaks' guilt in His Honor's death."

§

When he had finished, Marina posed a question. "I believe that no one will ever know of my husband's...lapse, but what of him? Will he be damned to the lowest hell?"

Michael lowered his eyes. "As I've said, I don't believe he died a traitor. But it's not for me or any mortal to judge him." His mouth tensed as he pursued the thought: who indeed could follow the turnings of the human heart or calculate the distance between heaven and hell? Sometimes it was a great gulf, at other times a mere blade's edge. "Father Zosimas would not have condemned him," he said.

Marina reached out, and let her hand cover his. "I thank you."

Michael rose. "Never mind that." He tried to swallow the lump of grief in his throat. "But—may I have the parchment? I think it's time we put an end to this." He extended his hand.

Marina pulled the folded document from her sleeve and gave it to him. She watched as he walked over to the brazier and dropped the parchment on the glowing coals.

Marina gasped, and Olympia slipped an arm around her shoulders. "This is the best thing to do." Flames sprung up around the page, and the two women fell silent as it curled, blackened, and vanished into ash and acrid smoke.

§

Later Olympia joined Michael downstairs, in the semi-darkness of the reception room. "You've given her hope," she said. "You've—"

He studied her joined hands in the flickering lamplight. He moved closer. "I wasn't lying."

"I know...I—" She appeared about to say something, but

386

hesitated.

"Is something wrong?" he asked.

"On the contrary," she said.

He watched the gleam of the soft light on her face, on the fine golden hairs above her mouth. She was smiling.

"My father has dismissed my would-be suitor," she said. "He heard some talk that the man takes bribes."

Michael laughed softly. "You can thank your teacher for that. And I believe it's true."

"No, my father does not countenance dishonesty. So you shouldn't judge him too harshly. He believes in all things honorable, but he's stubborn. If he knew about you— But he'll need to."

He approached and took her hands. "What are we going to do?"

Their eyes met, and she saw new life in them, new life, and something inexplicable. Here he was, like an army terrible with banners.

She pulled his hands toward her, and their lips touched. He was so close, and closer, as she dropped his hands, then drew her own around his head. He slipped an arm around her waist, and she rested against the wall.

"Oh!" she exclaimed, and wrested herself free. "I'm—"

He slammed his hand against the wall, and it came away bleeding. "I will never cause you to weep!" he said.

"But I'm not weeping," she said, now regarding his hand with the eyes of a physician.

"We need to be together," he said. "Do you see?"

"I do. But now we need to fix your hand. We'll get some water from the kitchen."

"I—I think I'd better go."

"Wait!" She took his injured hand and examined it, then dropped it and pulled a handkerchief from her sleeve. As she arranged it over his scraped knuckles and tied it, her white hands moved with the grace of doves. "Make sure you clean this out when you get home."

"My housekeeper will know what to do."

Without a word, they turned into the vestibule, towards the doors.

Michael regarded her. "So, what do we do now?"

She took his arm, but lowered her eyes. "We soldier on, and we hope for the best."

List of Characters

Alphabetical and by household / organization where appropriate.

Bartholomew, a farmer
   Cosmas, Bartholomew's son

Bishop of Cyzicus, a judge at the trial of Zosimas
Boian, a Bogomil Perfect, the mysterious outlander at Fr. Zosimas's trial

Michael Cerularius, Patriarch (chief bishop of the Church of Constantinople)
Isaac Comnenus, soldier, commander-in-chief of eastern armies and former employer of George
Cyril, subdeacon and assigned as assistant to Michael in the Patriarchal Library

Varangian Guard, Russo-Scandinavian bodyguards of the Emperor
   Ingvar, a Varangian
   Akolouthos, commander of Varangians

The Emperor's Household
   Constantine Monomachus, Emperor
   Zoe, Empress
   Augusta, the Emperor's young mistress
   Barbara, Empress Zoe's former maid, former mistress of
      Michael the Caulker

Symeon, Barbara's son

Nicetas Saponas, Rector, head of His Majesty's Household, a former soapmaker

Mark Saponas, son of Nicetas

Leo Syropoulos, *Kanikleios* (Custodian of the Imperial Inkstand)

Andronicus Acropolites, Court Physician

Lady Olympia Macrembolitissa, Acropolites's student and Michael's love interest

Basil Macrembolites, Lady Olympia's father

Irene Macrembolitissa, Lady Olympia's mother

Constantine Psellus, Emperor's First Secretary and head of the Faculty of Philosophy, at the state-run university

Luke, an eighteen-year-old shepherd, allegedly cousin to the grocer Peter of Serrhes. He has accused Father Zosimas of harassment and molestation.

Matthew, a novice at the Monastery of the Studion who also accuses Zosimas of harassment

Michael the Caulker, seized the throne after his uncle Emperor, Michael IV, died

Patzinaks

Metiga, a Patzinak and nephew of Kegen (war leader and head of Patzinaks)

Tirakh Khan, also leader of Patzinaks and Kegen's rival

Uzun, Metiga's half-brother

The Post

George Blachernites, Logothete of the Dromos, head of the Imperial Post, and Michael's superior

Eustathios Bourtzes, Agent of the Post and murder victim

Marina Bourtzes, Bourtzes's widow

Damien, the Bourtzes's servant

John Diogenes, Agent of the Post

Michael Taronites, Agent of the Post

Theodore Taronites, Michael's father and childhood friend of Father Zosimas

George, Michael Taronites's manservant

Theodosia, Michael Taronites's housekeeper

Stephen, George and Theodosia's son

Gregory Tripsychos, Agent of the Post and Bourtzes's rival for Marina

The Monastery of the Studion

The Abbot of the Monastery of the Studion

Jonas, a priestmonk and member of the Monastery of the Studion who accuses Zosimas of having a lover

Father Zosimas, a monk at the Monastery of the Studion and spiritual father of Michael Taronites

Naum Vladislavic, Father Zosimas's brother and *Hypostrategos* (lieutenant-general of the army of the Theme of Macedonia) and vice-

governor of the province
Mother Anastasia, sister of Fr. Zosimas

Peter of Serrhes, grocer who accused Zosimas of harassing his cousin, Luke

Susanna, an attendant of Augusta (the Emperor's mistress) who attempts to seduce Michael

Tornicius, rebel, blinded by Monomachus's order

Acknowledgements

Apparently, our mother began writing this book many years ago while living on the East Coast. She was a self-described recluse, and while she spoke animatedly about Byzantine history, she did not speak extensively about her writing.

Before she died, M.L. Jerinic self-published two novels, including the first volume in a proposed mystery series. After her sudden death, her husband, George Jerinic, found a nearly completed manuscript of a second mystery, Volume 2 in the series *A Byzantine Murder Mystery*.

Thanks to the efforts of Erik Pihel and Palamedes Publishing, this novel will reach a wide audience. We are immensely grateful for this support.

We also are grateful for the engaged community of readers across the country who have encouraged the author's work over the years.

All editing errors, historical or stylistic, are mine, and I beg your understanding. I do not have my mother's extensive knowledge of Byzantium, a lack which may influence the nuances and subtleties in these pages.

Maria Jerinic, June 2024

About the Author

M.L. Jerinic (1944-2021) was a reclusive writer, translator, and bibliophile who resided in North America. She was an avid reader with wide-ranging literary tastes. Despite her solitary habits, she enjoyed discussing all things bookish and historical.

She worked as a translator, book reviewer, and bookseller, and is the author of the epic, *The Sword of the Spirit: A Novel of Byzantium* and the mystery, *The Eunuch's Secret: A Byzantine Murder Mystery.*

M.L. Jerinic passed away suddenly on October 16, 2021. In addition to an extensive library, she left behind a nearly completed manuscript, *A Warrior's Death,* the second volume in the *Byzantine Murder Mystery* series. With support from her husband, George Jerinic, her daughters, Maria Jerinic and Katarina Jerinic, completed the manuscript edits and cover art, respectively.